Book and Cover Design by: AnnMarie Wyncoll

ISBN-13: 978-0-9956424-6-1 (paperback)
ISBN-13: 978-0-9956424-7-8 (ebook)

First paperback edition published in the
United Kingdom, November 2021

Published by: Begin-A-Book Independent Publishers
(www.beginabook.com)

***

Dedication

This book is dedicated to all the Chiari warriors who are dealing with this condition every day.

I hope this book gives you support, a voice and brings you comfort knowing you are not alone.

***

Acknowledgements

Thank you to the consultant who finally put all the pieces together and diagnosed my Chiari, without whom I would not be here today.

I would like to acknowledge all the staff at the neurocentre for their unwavering care and support on my journey.

My biggest thanks go to my family and close friends who have stood by me over the years from pre diagnosis to today. Your patience and understanding means the world and getting me to this point today has been very much a team effort....thank you.

Joanne xx

***

Chiari and Me - It's Not Just a Headache...

JOANNE ROBERTSON

***

Introduction

You have probably happened upon this book because you are one of the unlucky 1 in 1000 (approx.) people diagnosed with Chiari, or you know someone with Chiari and would like tips on how you can help them.

Through this book I want to give hope to Chiari sufferers and their families and, by also telling you about my journey before diagnosis, and then through treatment, give a voice to Chiari warriors out there who are struggling to be heard and maybe need reassurance that they are not alone.

Like me, you may never have heard of Chiari before your diagnosis, and you will be wondering what the heck it is. There are plenty of medical books and research papers out there to look at but not many books tell you how it really is, and how it's going to affect you and your life.

I have tried to be honest in this book, some of it is hard to read, God knows it was hard to write at times, but I wanted you to hear it from the perspective of someone living with Chiari. I've also included tips and advice that my family and I have picked up along the way to try and make your journey a little bit easier.

You will have been told no doubt that Chiari isn't curable, even with surgery, but the overriding message that I want you to take away from this book is **hope**. There is light at the end of the tunnel. This book will give you comfort in knowing that you're not alone, and will provide you with information and advice to help you get taken seriously, diagnosed quickly, and treated in good time. I also want it to bring comfort to your family and friends. What I have learnt about Chiari Malformation is that it affects everyone in your life, so they need to understand how your condition affects you, and each person is different. There are diverse classes, stages, associated problems etc, it can depend how long you've had it and to what extent, and if you've had any surgery. When I was first diagnosed with Chiari, I had never heard of it. By the time I saw my neurosurgeon it became clear I'd had it all my life. So many of the health issues I've experienced over the years can be attributed to the Chiari. It had always been in the background simmering away undetected, slowly taking hold and building in its ferocity.

After finally being diagnosed after ten years of struggle, closely followed by three brain surgeries in as many years, I'm still taking strong painkillers every single day. And every single day is a challenge.

But I am learning to adapt to my new normal and I will be forever grateful to be able to say that my journey isn't over …

and is to be continued...

***

The Diaries

***

Andrew

8th June 2018 - 2 days after decompression

I went to visit.

Joanne was down the far end of the ward. She didn't look well. She was complaining about her throat and that she couldn't swallow. The nurses gave her a cup of tea in a beaker with a spout. They said it would be good for her. But it wasn't. She kept coughing and choking and foaming at the mouth. Her head was bad she said. In fact, she pleaded with the nurses to 'put her down – I can't cope with this'. I remember the nurse joking that the bed would not go any lower. It wasn't funny.

Joanne's dad went home, and we agreed I should stay. I was concerned. Very concerned. I pulled a nurse to one side.

"Don't worry," she said, "Joanne's in good hands. Go home."

I didn't.

Sometime later another nurse arrived. A male nurse. He examined Joanne and said he wasn't happy with her. She was coughing up blood. He took her for an x-ray but by the time he brought her back she had deteriorated. They moved her to the High Dependency Unit and en-route she vomited.

The x-rays were back. Joanne had a large shadow on one lung. In the background someone said she should've been nil by mouth after her operation. They took me to one side. Joanne had aspiration pneumonia, they said. She needed to go to intensive care (ITU).

I was taken to the family room in ITU and told to wait, that someone would come and tell me what was happening. I waited.

An hour and a half later I was still waiting. I decided to find out what was going on. I located some doors and pressed a buzzer. Eventually someone came out to see me. They apologised, explained they didn't know I was there.

It had been over two hours since I'd last seen Joanne. And I knew nothing.

I was allowed into intensive care to see her. Briefly. On the wall was a board detailing all her stats. They were coded like traffic lights, red, amber, and green. Virtually all of Joanne's numbers were red. I searched frantically until I found a couple that were green. At least that was something.

I stayed at the hospital that night although I was only allowed to see Joanne for a few minutes. I looked at the board again.

Still mostly red but I thought I saw more green.

And that was my life day after day. Visiting Joanne, watching that board, praying for amber and green to overtake the red.

It was all we talked about as a family and every little sign of improvement was something we clung to.

Desperately.

***

Joanne

2018

It was to be ten years before I was diagnosed with Chiari. It began with headaches, but I was getting more and more of these. They were unusual, coming on abruptly without warning. Every sudden movement such as coughing or laughing was agony.

One of my earliest memories was the summer when I was going to be a bridesmaid for my cousin. I had never been a bridesmaid, so I was absolutely over the moon and honoured to have been asked. As I recall everything went okay, we got ready at my cousins and then went to the ceremony. At the reception there was the usual round of photographs followed by a lovely meal and the speeches. I was so happy and had no warning of what was about to happen.

The party began and it wasn't long before my favourite Bon Jovi song was played. I grabbed Andrew's hand and we made our way towards the dancefloor, when suddenly I experienced a crippling, crushing pain in my head. I was going to fall to the floor – I knew it – so I grabbed harder onto Andrew to keep me upright. My mum saw what was happening and encouraged me to sit down, though she didn't understand.

"You're a bridesmaid," she said, "don't make a fuss."

I sat for a while, but the pain didn't shift, and I knew I needed to lie down. Andrew and I were staying at the hotel where the reception was being held so we made our excuses and left early. Back in the hotel room I simply collapsed onto the bed, the pain almost unbearable.

These episodes continued and as time went on, I found the simplest of tasks, such as getting up and ready for the day, exhausted me. I thought that maybe I was straining my head and neck when I was doing my hair and makeup and perhaps that was the cause. I'd have to lie down mid-way through getting ready and rest until it passed.

Other things changed. Having suffered with back problems since my mid-twenties, the usual grumbles or twinges didn't concern me but by the end of 2014, the pain in my back was extreme. I found myself unable to walk for any distance and was beginning to take time off work.

My as yet unknown illness was starting to take its toll.

***

Andrew

10th June 2018

Joanne had been moved into her own room and seemed more stable. In fact, she began to complain so I knew the signs were good. We had finally turned a corner.

The tube in her throat had caused some damage so her voice was high-pitched. It sounded strange to my ears, but I have never been more relieved to hear someone speak. After a time, she was moved back onto the main ward, but she couldn't do anything. It was like the operation had robbed her of everything she'd ever learned. We had to start at the beginning, teaching her how to use a spoon and fork. Every day I offered encouragement, told her how well she was doing, but in reality, I was crumbling.

I used to leave her on occasions to get some rest and go to the canteen but that was all. During those moments I allowed myself to let my guard down and simply feel, be at one with myself.

In many ways these times were the most frightening as I experienced every single emotion possible. I was worried, concerned, heartbroken, helpless, low…but that was nothing compared to what Jo was going through and I knew I had to be strong. There was no other choice.

I quickly learned to be Joanne's voice, to tell those around her when things weren't right, when I wasn't happy. I knew Joanne better than anyone and whilst I didn't want to make a fuss, I knew when she wasn't okay, and I had to make myself heard. Some days that was tough.

Whilst she was in ITU, Joanne had not been sleeping properly, almost as if she had to recover from the surgery before she could relax. When she was finally back on the main ward, she did little else but sleep and I didn't know what to do for her. Did I stay in case she woke up? Did I go and get some rest so that I could be there for her when she was better? Did I need to worry about her sleeping all the time?

The questions and the internal torture were endless.

Joanne was surrounded by suction pipes and machinery. One day she was encouraged to have some physio on her chest. To me it looked like they were jumping up and down on her and I panicked. She was given a device, a tube to blow into so that she could inflate a ball. It exhausted her. Joanne had nothing left.

At this point all I could do was sit silently by and hope.

***

Joanne

2015

The back pain had become so debilitating that I knew I needed medical advice. I went to the doctor who examined me before prescribing strong painkillers.

"One of those things" he said, "something to just live with."

I remember thinking I didn't want to put up with this. I hated not being in control of my health and couldn't believe that painkillers were my only option. I was in my forties, but I felt like an old woman. I made a decision. I would only take a minimal number of painkillers so that if the pain increased, I could take more. That way I would have some kind of control.

At the beginning of 2015 I realised that the pains in my head were getting worse and not only that, the dizzy spells were on the increase. I went back to the doctor who suggested I needed some physiotherapy.

My back, head and dizziness were, he said, all connected.

This sounded plausible so I went home and awaited an appointment. The day of my physiotherapy treatment arrived. I was getting ready to leave when once again I was hit by dizziness, but this time my vision blurred. I sat down on the bed waiting for it to pass, but it didn't. I realised I would have to cancel my appointment. I couldn't even get up let alone have therapy.

For a few days after this I was off work sick. The dizziness was horrendous, my back was killing me, and the headaches were with me every hour of every day. I called the doctor who prescribed Tramadol to relax my muscles. It didn't work. The headaches would not budge, the pain was unbearable, I couldn't sit, stand, or move. There was no relief.

I called the doctor again, but I couldn't get an appointment. The only way I could be seen was to go to the surgery and 'sit and wait' until a doctor was free. It took three hours. Three hours of absolute torture. I couldn't find comfort anywhere, so in the end I asked the receptionist if I could return to my car and wait – at least there I could recline the seat and lie down. I couldn't, I was told. If I left the surgery, I would lose my place in the 'sit and wait' queue.

The torture continued.

***

Andrew

2015

My earliest memories of Joanne having problems was about three years before her diagnosis. She was experiencing severe headaches most mornings which I thought could simply be stress related. But then she showed other symptoms – the most concerning of which was the fact she choked on her food. It didn't matter what she ate, even something smooth like a yoghurt, would cause her to choke as she struggled to swallow.

When Joanne first described her pain to me, I figured I understood. It was a headache. We all have headaches, but as I watched her deteriorating, I knew that I had absolutely no idea what she was going through. The endless round of doctor's appointments began.

At first, I didn't think it was serious. The doctor advised self-help remedies such as drinking less coffee, avoiding stress, going to physiotherapy… but nothing helped.

I supported Joanne with all these things, yet it became farcical as time after time the remedies failed. The doctors simply had no answers. Joanne had got to the point where she needed to hold onto a wall or furniture when the pain hit to prevent herself from collapsing. Rarely did we see the same GP (doctor) twice and every time she had to explain her symptoms, over and over again.

I still don't think I realised how bad she had got. Joanne had started eating alone in our bedroom because the choking was making her self-conscious. She didn't want me and the boys to see it. I listened out for her, for any sign of a problem but it wasn't until we were on a family holiday, I realised just how poorly she was. She choked at every single mealtime and the consistency of the food was irrelevant. I started to feel scared and for the first time considered that maybe this was something serious after all.

A few weeks later Joanne and I went on a spa break, just the two of us. By this time, she had started experiencing episodes of compromised breathing during her sleep, to the point where she would actually stop. At home we often slept in separate rooms as Joanne found resting hard – not helped by my snoring – but when we were on the spa break, I saw first-hand what was happening. She would stop breathing for what felt like an eternity, and then wake, gasping for breath. I was frightened. Beyond frightened.

From that day on I watched her like a hawk.

***

Joanne

2015

Eventually I was seen. The doctor prescribed Naproxen, Omeprazole and repeat Tramadol. He also requested blood tests and x-rays on my Sacro-iliac joints. He told me that if there was any sign of inflammation he would refer me to rheumatology - if not then I would be seen at the spinal clinic and offered acupuncture. Despondent and still in agony, I went home.

The bloods came back a few days later and there was no sign of inflammation. This meant I was sent to the spinal clinic. Here it was suggested I had a bulging disc in my spine but would need an MRI (Magnetic Resonance Imaging) scan to formally diagnose. In the meantime, I was given acupuncture which did sometimes help. Other days though, I could be left in even worse pain for a couple of days afterwards.

When the MRI results came back, I remember feeling relieved.

I genuinely thought this would provide the answers we needed. A diagnosis and the right treatment.

The results showed several things: enlarged facet joints, shortened pedicules and lateral recess stenosis. I had no idea what any of it meant but it seemed I had got lucky with a triple whammy of problems. Not.

Back surgery, the doctor advised, was the best option and so I was referred to the neurocentre. I began to feel like a ping pong ball bouncing from one department to another with little in the way of solutions. They still didn't know what was wrong, but the pain was indescribable, and waiting for one department then another and then another …

Somehow, I managed to go back to work but I was on a whole host of painkillers. The phrase 'being hit by a ton of bricks' came to mind and it was all I could do to survive the day. As soon as I got home, I would collapse on the sofa and that would be it. The constant level of pain I was experiencing was exhausting but I knew that if I was going to have surgery, I needed to keep working so I could have the time off when I needed it.

This continued until the August when I was finally seen at the neurocentre, a few months after the initial referral. They reviewed my MRI and confirmed I had a narrowing of the spinal canal at L4/5 with shortened pedicules. I was told there were no surgical options, and that conservative management was the way forward. Painkillers and physiotherapy. I was back to square one.

Around this time, I began to have problems with my throat. It was sore for weeks and I started to cough up blood. Another trip to the doctor who diagnosed glandular fever. More blood tests. More x-rays. More clear test results. No diagnosis. Nothing to find. Another mystery.

Then, in the summer of 2015, everything changed. Suddenly and unexpectedly, I lost my mum. I was floored. My two sons were in the midst of O and A Levels respectively and they needed my support. I couldn't afford to worry about my own health - not when our family was grieving, and my boys were at such a crucial life point. It would have been selfish.

For the next two years I lived on autopilot. I kept taking the painkillers to get through each day, I showed up for work and for my family … rinse and repeat.

It was an endless cycle: work, home, bed, sleep, reprise.

***

Joanne

March 2017

Things deteriorated.

We had been invited to the evening wedding reception for one of Andrew's friends. This was taking place in Manchester. Having checked into the hotel in which we were staying, we joined some other friends for a meal in town before going on to the wedding reception. To begin with I felt okay. I managed to eat my meal and even treated myself to a cocktail but suddenly the pressure and pain began to build in my head. I couldn't speak properly. Every time I tried to make myself heard, I thought my head was going to explode. Thinking fresh air would help, I left the table and sat outside for a while. Andrew joined me.

The fresh air didn't help so slowly, we walked back to the hotel. In our room I had a lie down before getting ready for the evening reception. Though I managed this, I couldn't shake the nausea and fuzziness in my head, or the constant pain.

We arrived at the reception early and it was still quiet. We chose a table near the back of the room, against a wall and well away from the dancefloor and speakers. I needed as much distance from the noise as possible. I lasted about an hour. The pain in my head continued to worsen and, thinking I may simply be dehydrated, I drank only water and lemonade, but nothing helped. After just over sixty minutes I excused myself and returned to our room where I lay as still as I could in the darkness.

The pain remained with me, there was no respite and so, a couple of days later I managed to get another doctor's appointment. I explained how painful my head had been and how it had affected me but again, this was a different GP who I'd not seen before. He thought it was my eyes and told me to get them tested. Oh, and to drink less coffee.

OMG. I was literally banging my head against a brick wall.

By this time, I was having regular physiotherapy through work. The therapist would massage my neck and shoulders as these had become very tight and tense which, she suggested, could well be the cause of the head pain. Though I had numerous sessions and several attempts to loosen my muscles, it made no difference to the agony in my head. It wouldn't go away.

One of the girls at work recommended a chiropractor. I was willing to try anything, so I made an appointment. The first couple of times I did get some relief in my neck and shoulders. The chiropractor explained that as my neck muscles were so tight, she would manipulate them to loosen them a little and then use strong tape to keep the muscles in place. It sounds bizarre now, but I was desperate.

Like I say, the first couple of times I went with it, persevered with the taping, and was convinced it would work. The third time I was in agony for days afterwards. I was recommended to another chiropractor, and I figured why not? I was so distressed by the awful head and neck pains, it no longer mattered what treatment was offered. I would take it.

I now know that seeing a chiropractor was one of the worst things I could possibly have done. When I think of how the second specialist manipulated my neck, it makes me feel sick.

If you have a Chiari, you should not see a chiropractor. Ever. He had a gun like device that he used to 'knock my neck and spine joints back into alignment'.

We had no way of knowing that my brain had prolapsed and that in fact, this procedure was incredibly dangerous for me. I trusted the experts. He was confident that this treatment would work. It didn't. All it did was exacerbate my existing symptoms and bring on new ones.

Oddly I am grateful that it didn't help because if it had done, I would have continued with the treatment. The manipulation would almost certainly have had a devastating outcome.

May 2017

A weird thing happened. I lost my voice suddenly without warning and it didn't come back for five days. There was no sore throat or cough, I just couldn't speak. As I wasn't unwell, I continued going to work but I couldn't take any calls. Instead, I put a sticky label on my top stating that I had lost my voice and helped visitors to the department as much as I could. It was an interesting few days. On the sixth day, as suddenly as it had gone, my voice returned. Though we were relieved, I think

Andrew was a little disappointed. He had, he said, enjoyed the peace and quiet.

Shortly after this, Andrew and I were invited to a masquerade ball. I was so excited. I had always dreamed of going to a ball, wearing a lovely dress, and dancing with Andrew in his dashing tuxedo. We both embraced planning our costumes and selecting our masks and, on the day of the ball, we were greeted by pipers on arrival, who played us into dinner. It was amazing. The tables were beautifully set, there were gorgeous dresses everywhere I looked, smartly dressed men in dinner suits and so many masks.

We were seated on a round table, which sounds trivial, but it meant I didn't have to twist my neck all the time. Everything was going well. We were having a fantastic evening.

The meal arrived. The starter…no problem but when the main meal came and I started to eat, I choked. I was embarrassed. I tried to be discreet, but tears were streaming down my face. I abandoned my meal.

The dessert was cheesecake. I managed to eat the soft top part and even joked with my friend that I'd live on cheesecake topping, but I was so fed up. I had wanted to eat my meal – all of it.

Later, there was a charity auction. I bid on a love seat for the garden but narrowly missed out. Andrew's face was a picture as he watched my hand shoot up. I was having so much fun. For one night I almost felt normal.

As the raffle ended, (in which we won the star prize - a hamper of luxury food – oh, the irony!), I felt a headache brewing so took my usual trip outside for fresh air. I was angry, frustrated and in pain. I wanted to dance with my husband and enjoy the evening with our friends, instead of which I was searching for a non-existent quiet corner in an attempt to find relief.

It was hopeless. Once again, we made our apologies and once again, we left. Early.

July 2017

We were preparing to go on holiday to Lanzarote. I decided to get my nails done and went to my usual salon. All was well when I arrived but, as I reached up to hang my jacket on a hook, I experienced the worst crushing pain in my head. I was dizzy, I couldn't stand and had to hold onto the wall to prevent me from collapsing to the floor.

My nail technician was shocked. Having a customer almost pass out was not something she'd been expecting. Once I was able, she helped me to sit down and gave me a glass of water. The pain gradually subsided but the sickness, nausea and thick head remained. I was also unable to move my neck. At this point I was frightened to say the least.

I had also been having more trouble eating. I'd been choking more often than not so had switched to softer foods with a smooth texture. By this time, I was feeling so unwell, that I had taken to eating my evening meal in the bedroom. It was quieter and more relaxed, plus I didn't want Andrew and the boys to see me choking all the time.

When we got to Lanzarote we began eating as a family again and it became apparent to Andrew how much I had deteriorated. He made me promise to get my eating and choking issues checked out as soon as we returned home. I said I would.

Even though the physiotherapy had not really helped, I found myself missing the release of some of the tension around my neck. I decided to book a massage at the hotel spa, thinking it would be good for me, relaxing even. It left me in agony. I couldn't lie comfortably on the sun lounger for two whole days, but Andrew and I laughed it off.

"No pain, no gain" we said, expecting it to settle down.

As the holiday progressed, other symptoms appeared until one day, I found myself unable to climb into the minibus taxi. My right leg just gave up. It didn't collapse but there was no strength in it, none whatsoever. With the help of the boys and my left leg, we finally managed to get me into the taxi. Yet again my body was failing me, and I had no idea why.

On my return home I did as I had promised my family and went to the doctor about my choking. I also needed to discuss my HRT (hormone replacement therapy), so I went with the intention of discussing both. I wasn't overly worried at that point - I figured it was another 'one of those things' that I was so used to hearing.

Knowing I had more than one symptom to talk about, I made sure to book a double appointment. When I walked in, and the GP asked how she could help I said I was having trouble choking on my food and could we review my HRT medications as it didn't seem to be helping with my hot flushes. We subsequently learned that one of the symptoms of Chiari is not being able to regulate your body temperature, but we didn't know I had Chiari at that point.

The doctor immediately said we needed to leave the HRT issue for now and deal with the choking. She asked me lots of questions about how often, what type of food, what it was like and seemed genuinely concerned. A referral to the gastroenterology department at the hospital was suggested and I balked at the thought of more appointments and more tests, so I asked if it was necessary.

Yes, she stated, it was.

The next thing I knew, the doctor began to consult an information sheet on throat cancer and asked if I had any other symptoms. I explained about the head pains and nausea. She told me to try not to worry and that it was a good sign that I wasn't losing weight. Try not to worry? Easy for her to say!

It took another two weeks before I received the appointment from the gastroenterology department. Two weeks of interminable worry. Whilst I knew an endoscopy was my only choice, I found myself absolutely dreading it. I had a friend who'd been through one before and described it as an 'awful experience'.

The day of the appointment arrived, and I was taken into a room by a lovely nurse who saw how nervous I was.

She was very understanding and offered me sedation, though she said it would delay me being able to go home. I told her to give me all the sedation they could and watched as she wrote 'lots of sedation' on the form.

It obviously worked as I don't remember the procedure at all. Result.

After the endoscopy I had a doze before being woken up with a cup of tea and some biscuits. Shortly afterwards the doctor arrived and explained they had found nothing untoward. It was, he said, oesophageal reflux and heartburn and he would contact my GP to prescribe regular antacids. I asked if these conditions would cause me to choke and he assured me they would so as ever, I trusted what he said. I left happy and relieved. There was nothing sinister going on.

September 2017

Over the summer I had decided to start up a business selling skincare products. I knew that both boys would be away from home at university, and I wanted something to do with any spare time I might have. I'd always fancied the idea of being self-employed and this ticked all the boxes, so I threw myself into it. I went to meetings every couple of weeks where I met loads of like-minded women. These meetings were great fun, and I would leave feeling motivated and upbeat. I felt this was going to be a really positive business and experience.

In September of 2017 I did a skincare pamper at my neighbour's house. Everything was going well; I had completed the pamper session but suddenly the room began to get noisy. The guests were chatting and laughing, and I found myself having to raise my voice. Then I noticed I was feeling dizzy.

At the same time, one of the ladies asked if I could do a foot pamper but I knew there was no way I'd be able to bend over to complete it. I had been down this road of dizziness so many times before. I was embarrassed to give the real reason though, so I told her I had a dodgy knee. In the end her friend helped her, and they had a great time.

By now I was really struggling with the noise and couldn't wait for the evening to be over. When it was time to pack up though, I was hit by a blinding, crushing pain in my head, and realised I could not move it at all. I rang Andrew and he came to pick me up. I felt awful, not only because of the excruciating pain but because I felt I had let the hostess down. I thought I should have been more upbeat, more entertaining, but I couldn't.

Later that month I attended a conference and recognition event for my little business. The journey down wasn't too bad. I sat in the front of the car and was quite comfortable. When we arrived though, there was opportunity to grab a coffee and chat and live musicians were playing, which made for an extremely noisy welcome. Whilst I was loving the atmosphere, I could feel the pressure in my head starting to build. Again. I couldn't wait to sit down.

Entering the main hall, I felt so dizzy that I could barely walk to my table. Luckily, I was able to position myself facing the stage so at least I wouldn't have to twist my head around to see what was going on. We got to lunchtime, and I managed the light buffet by eating only the softer options and drinking plenty of water.

I was able to talk to the ladies either side of me but only if I moved my whole body to face them – they must have thought I was very odd.

Between the day and evening events there was opportunity to relax. Myself and my friends weren't staying over which meant we didn't have rooms to rest in. Instead, we found some comfy chairs in the foyer where it was nice and quiet. By the time the evening's festivities began I was feeling quite tired but excited. This was going to be a good night.

Prior to the event I'd been experiencing a lot of hot flushes and episodes of sweating, alternated with chills and periods of being unable to get warm. Being of a certain age we presumed it was menopause related. I tried everything to regulate my temperature, but nothing worked. It had got so bad that I would take a spare t-shirt with me wherever I went.

During the evening, we were offered the opportunity to meet the founder of the company we worked for and have our photograph taken with her. I remember standing in line and waiting for about 20-30 minutes, getting hotter and hotter as each second ticked by. My make-up was melting off me, I was literally dripping. The friends I was with were fine – it was just me.

As we got nearer to the front of the line, I bottled it. There was no way I wanted to meet someone I admired whilst sweating like I was. I pulled out of the line and went to sit back down.

After a bit of chatting and music, the hot buffet was served. I was only on my second mouthful when I started to choke. I thought it was the texture, so I tried some other bits, but it was no use. I couldn't continue to eat.

The now familiar blinding pain was engulfing my head to the point I was clutching at it. My friends helped me out to the quietness of the foyer where I found a seat in a corner. I must have stayed out in that foyer for at least two hours. There was nothing I could do. My friend was driving, and it was too far for Andrew to come and collect me – though he did offer.

My friends kept coming to check on me and brought me drinks of water, but I insisted I was fine. I didn't want to ruin their evening too. Plus, it felt trivial to say I had a headache, but it was so much more than that. The pain was crippling.

Through all the tests and visits to the doctor nothing had been found that could explain my symptoms, so I had started to believe I was going mad.

And, that this was something I was just going to have to learn to live with.

It was to be only a few weeks later when I had yet another episode of coughing, choking and excruciating pain. I was at a friend's house and ended up collapsing into a chair. Andrew came to collect me. Yet another evening ruined.

The pain, which was brought on by choking, coughing, sneezing, laughing, hiccups… in fact, pretty much anything – was becoming more severe and frighteningly, occurring with increasing regularity.

***

Joanne
Friday 30th March 2018

I collapsed.

I remember being sat on the sofa with Andrew and we were looking at something funny on his phone. I laughed out loud and then collapsed into him. The pressure in my head was immense and I couldn't lift it back up. Nor could I move.

Andrew phoned the out of hours doctor and the next thing I remember is being in Accident and Emergency, trying to describe what had happened. The memories are a little fuzzy, but I do know the doctor referred to 'red flag symptoms' and that she would be keeping me in for tests.

That night I had a CT scan, which, predictably, revealed nothing. The following day I was sent for a lumbar puncture to rule out meningitis.

(I have since learned that a lumbar puncture can be dangerous for Chiari patients unless you have had surgery for decompression. Obviously, we didn't know this at the time).

The lumbar puncture was negative. No meningitis.

By now I had become extremely sensitive to light and sound, so spent much of the day with the curtains drawn around me. I lost count of the number of times I had to explain to a well-meaning nurse or domestic why I had the curtains drawn when they came to open them. I was lucky though. The other ladies in the bay with me were lovely and didn't mind keeping the blinds shut or the television on low. Soon they became my voice when anyone tried to open my curtains.

By the Monday I had extreme nausea, severe head pains and slurred speech. I was that unsteady on my feet that I had to use a commode rather than walk to the loo. After a couple of days on the ward a lovely consultant came to see me on her rounds. Again, I had to explain what had brought me in and what my symptoms were. She ordered an MRI scan, and I had a feeling she knew what she was looking for.

The next day I was eating my lunch when the registrar came to see me with a copy of the scan result. It confirmed I had a Chiari Malformation with a tonsillar descent of 3cm below the craniocervical junction extending to the bottom of C2 with a significant compression. There was also distortion of the 4th ventricle. I had no idea what any of that meant.

When I questioned the registrar, she said it was something to do with my brain and that a referral had been sent to the neurocentre.

Had she heard of this before? I asked.

No, she admitted, she hadn't.

Later I saw the consultant, the one who had requested the MRI and asked if she had heard of Chiari Malformation. She had. She'd recognised my symptoms and knew that if it was Chiari it would show on an MRI.

I couldn't believe it.

Finally.

Finally, we knew what was wrong with me. The relief was immense, but then I learned what was to come.

> ~ *A note here to that wonderful consultant to whom I am forever indebted. I am so incredibly grateful that she recognised the symptoms and after ten years, took the right steps* ~

When the specialist from the neurocentre arrived, he explained a little about Chiari and what it meant for me. He said that I was highly likely to need brain surgery and drew me a diagram on a piece of paper which I still have to this day (see following page).

He explained that my notes and scan results had been sent to the neurocentre and there was to be an MDT (multi-disciplinary team) meeting to discuss the next steps and treatment.

His advice? Rest and relax for the weekend and he would see me again on Monday. And try not to do anything that might bring on the head pain.

I rang Andrew in tears. I was terrified. I had literally just been told that my brain was hanging out of the bottom of my skull and pressing on my spinal column - I had no idea that this was even possible.

Andrew told me not to panic, that he was on his way to visit. I asked him to bring my dad too.

When they arrived, I showed them the picture and explained what little I knew. We asked the nurse if she could give us any more information, but she had not come across this before either. The diagram the specialist had left me with was as much a fascination to her as it was to us.

So, there wasn't much to do for a few days. Sit and wait. Again. I tried not to google it, but quickly found there wasn't much information anyway.

I attempted to relax over the weekend. The specialist had suggested that I might go straight to the neurocentre after the MDT, so my husband and sons arranged to bring my dogs down to the front door of the hospital to visit. At this point I had no idea when I would be home to be with them again. Andrew took me down in a wheelchair. I remember the dogs being more interested in the wheelchair than seeing me, but it did me the power of good to have them there. Even for such a short time.

Though I tried not to worry – everything was out of my hands in any case – I couldn't help becoming concerned when I developed a new symptom. I swallowed some juice but instead of going down into my stomach, it came straight back out through my nose in a steady flow. This freaked me out.

Monday came and the events of the past few days had begun to sink in. I was told though, that the results of the MDT hadn't been received yet, so they were going to discharge me, and I was to await a call from the neurocentre. I was put onto Amitriptyline to help with any nerve pain, and I remember the next day feeling dopey. I also found my right arm and left leg were heavy and sore and on top of that I had severe nausea, no appetite, head pain, fatigue, dizziness…in fact, I felt drunk. Whenever I moved, I had to use the wall to steady myself.

Two days later and we still hadn't heard from the hospital, so Andrew rang the neurocentre. It took a while as he was passed from one department to another but eventually, we discovered that my referral had been sent to the wrong department.

They assured me it would be resolved and, sure enough, I received an appointment for the neurocentre on the 8th of May.

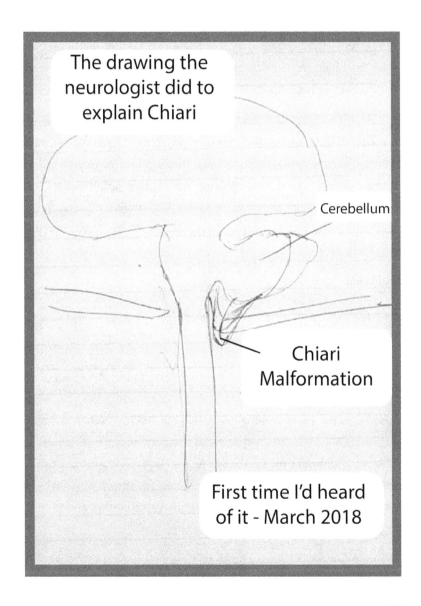

April 2018

Throughout April I continued to have problems. My head was muzzy and my whole body was sore. The pain around the back of my head was getting increasingly worse and I couldn't talk on the phone for more than half an hour. After thirty minutes I would feel so unwell that I'd have to hang up.

I gradually became more and more isolated. Often, I didn't feel up to seeing friends, and on the occasions when I did have visitors, they had no idea what to say. After a while they stopped ringing or calling round. Though I am certain the drugs weren't helping with how I felt, the pharmacist who reviewed me at the GP surgery advised me to stick with them. I was currently taking dihydrocodeine, amitriptyline and paracetamol.

And bonus…

I was developing yet more new symptoms.

My right arm had started twitching at the elbow and I had a constant dull pain down to the knuckles, yet my hand was freezing cold. I started wearing fingerless gloves all day.

I also noticed I was struggling to catch my breath sometimes, and then at other times I would have repeated bouts of hiccups. The pain in my head would wake me up at night and on several occasions, I would realise I'd been sick in my mouth and that my throat was burning. Like something was stuck. I took indigestion medication and tried to sleep sitting up.

The next few weeks passed so slowly, every day a kind of haze. We didn't know how I would be after the operation so I tried to get myself organised and make sure Andrew knew where everything was should the worst happen. Tensions were high. Andrew said he felt helpless and hated that things were out of his control.

One time we had an argument. We were in the utility room, and I shouted at him. My legs went from underneath me, and I collapsed to the floor. Simply because I shouted. This was crazy.

The days were fast becoming unbearable.

I was desperate for a treatment plan and, if I needed an operation, I wanted this to happen sooner rather than later.

Every morning I awoke with severe head pain, and didn't feel remotely refreshed. Something as simple as washing my hair would wipe me out for at least a couple of hours.

During this time, I had a couple of particularly horrendous episodes of crushing head pain. The first was when I bent to fill the washing machine. The second was whilst straining on the loo. Both episodes left me feeling drained, exhausted, unable to think straight and I couldn't string any words together.

I made myself go to the hairdressers. I wanted to try to do something normal even though I felt very unwell. It hurt to raise my voice over the sound of the hairdryers.

Andrew had taken me, so I didn't have to worry about driving. We decided to go for a bite to eat as we hadn't been getting out much, but I felt that lightheaded and nauseous, I ate very little, and we were soon heading home where I went straight to bed.

I was also developing pain through my neck and into my ears. Chiari really is the gift that keeps on giving.

I was so frustrated that I couldn't do simple things with my husband. To me, every moment we could spend together was vital. We didn't know what the outcome of my treatment or surgery would be.

With little information readily available, I joined a couple of Chiari groups on social media. One scared me to death, so I left almost as soon as I joined, another though was very helpful and supportive. A few people said they'd taken a list of questions with them to their appointment, and a list of their symptoms. This, I thought, was a good idea.

(See Resources Page at the end of the book for details of this and other groups I have found beneficial).

I remember it was sunny the day before my appointment, so Andrew and I sat in the back garden and made a note of all my symptoms. It was quite a list. Bizarrely I was still worried that the neurosurgeon would either not believe me or dismiss my symptoms as 'one of those things'. I was bracing myself to be told I needed physiotherapy or to drink less coffee.

Thankfully, I could not have been more wrong.

***

Andrew

Friday 30th March 2018

When Joanne collapsed, I rushed her to accident and emergency. By this time, I knew we were dealing with something out of the ordinary, but I had no clue what.

At the hospital I put my faith in the medical team. I prayed they would figure out what was wrong and then how to help her. Joanne was seen by a very young keen doctor who took time to talk through all of Joanne's symptoms with her. More tests followed. The young doctor said she'd spotted a few 'red flags' so she ordered a head CT (computed tomography) scan and a lumbar puncture. She wanted to rule out meningitis.

Though she was young, this was the first doctor we had seen who was trying to put all the pieces together and get a diagnosis. I will forever be grateful for the time and care that doctor gave and, as a result, Joanne was finally diagnosed. She had Chiari.

At first, I wasn't too worried. Joanne explained what little she knew to her dad and me and we felt relief that eventually she could be treated. I could tell though that Joanne was scared and in shock and knowing how important it was to keep her calm, that became my focus.

Joanne was admitted and, on the ward, I spoke to the doctor and nurses. They told me that Chiari was not a serious brain condition and was easy to fix. Little did I know just how wrong they were, and that this would turn out to be the biggest piece of misinformation ever.

Now that we had a diagnosis, things happened very quickly. I was shocked at the speed in fact. Joanne had joined an online Chiari support group and had read that many people struggled to explain to a specialist just how ill they were. Some, she told me, were left in tears of despair after being refused surgery or treatment. At least, I consoled, we were not in that position.

Joanne's first appointment at the neurocentre arrived and we armed ourselves with a list of her symptoms and how it was affecting her. We thought we might have to do battle again, but the surgeon could not have been more understanding. After reviewing Joanne's scans and showing us where the problem was, he commented on his surprise that she was still here. That she had survived this far. I explained to the consultant that we had tried to get treatment for years, but that Joanne had been continuously misdiagnosed.

It was at this point I realised exactly how serious this was and what a bad state Joanne was in. Nevertheless, the neurosurgeon reassured me he could help and that whilst the Chiari could not be permanently cured or fixed, he could release the decompression somewhat which would hopefully pause her symptoms.

She would, he said, not get any worse.

By now the Chiari malformation was affecting Joanne's breathing and swallowing. The surgeon said he needed to operate sooner rather than later, but he was due to go on holiday. He promised to schedule her surgery to be his first when he returned. If though, he reassured, her condition deteriorated, then another surgeon could do the operation as an emergency. I promised to let the neurocentre know if this happened, took Joanne home, made her comfortable and prayed she wouldn't deteriorate any further over the next two weeks.

When it came to the pre-op clinic at the neurocentre, I had to leave the room. The operation was being discussed in detail with Joanne so that she knew what to expect, but it was far from what I understood it to be. I'd read up on the operation and thought it would be an orthopaedic type of procedure involving vertebrae and bones, but in fact, it really was about Joanne's brain. The specialist nurse began expanding on what would happen and I couldn't cope. I felt sick, faint, and terrified. Thus, I had to leave the room.

I'm not proud of that. It was awful leaving Joanne to hear all of that by herself, but I knew that if I'd stayed, she would have been more worried about me than the details of her operation – because that's the kind of person Joanne is.

On the day of Joanne's operation, I was extremely nervous. When the love of your life is facing brain surgery, your stomach churns, and your mind races.

What will be the outcome? What is the worst that can happen? What if something goes wrong?

Joanne was incredible that day. She was so matter of fact when she reassured me everything would be fine and that she had to have this operation because then her life would be saved. I have never been prouder of her than I was that day.

If I could give one piece of advice to family or friends of the patient, it would simply be this:

Remember, your loved one is in the hands of experts.

***

Joanne

Tuesday 8th May 2018

Andrew and I arrived at the neurocentre for my long-awaited appointment. Today we were to find out exactly what was wrong with me.

The consultant was lovely, warm, and smiley. I immediately felt at ease. He asked how I had been, but it wasn't long before he turned his monitor around so that we could see my scan pictures. It was very clear, he said, that I had a significant Chiari malformation, and that surgery was required. Sooner rather than later. The scan told him everything. He didn't even look at my long list of symptoms.

Having had progressively worsening Chiari symptoms for many years, I had reached the point that whenever I strained, coughed, sneezed, or bent down I was in danger of collapsing. This, along with the choking episodes meant we were out of time. I needed surgical intervention.

The consultant explained that surgery was not a cure but would 'pause' my symptoms at the point of surgery so that I shouldn't continue to deteriorate. I didn't like the idea of it not being a cure, but I knew there was no choice to be made if I wanted a chance at some quality of life. I was also ready to take any help I could get!

I was in danger of serious complications from my Chiari and its resultant compression, so the consultant advised surgery for decompression, sooner rather than later.

The surgery is done under general anaesthetic. In a straightforward decompression surgery, a cut is made at the back of the head and neck and the skin and muscles are pulled back to allow the neurosurgeon to remove a small part of the base of the skull. Sometimes part of the top two vertebrae are removed as well, and sometimes the dura (which is the membrane covering the brain) is opened and a patch sewn in to make it bigger.

Before the operation I was told I would meet a specialist Chiari nurse who would go through everything in detail and answer any questions. Before I knew it, my surgery had been booked in for the 6th of June. Ten years to get here and now it was crazy how fast it was happening.

The day after that appointment I had a collapse. I had been numb since leaving hospital with the diagnosis as I'd tried to absorb everything, but that morning, the day after the consultant's appointment, it finally sunk in I was about to have brain surgery. Someone would be cutting into the back of my head and working on my brain.

I spent part of that day in tears and part of it asking my mum to look after me from her place in heaven. I talked to my mum all the time and I wanted her there with me in the only way I knew how.

My mind was all over the place. I could hardly eat and began to overthink even the smallest of things.

I soon discovered that because Chiari is not widely known, the information online varied hugely which triggered all kinds of negative thoughts. I have since learned to be careful what groups and websites I visit, and I would recommend sticking to sites that are regulated and official. The information provided by these sites will be the most accurate.

Back in my Facebook group, it was suggested that I make a list of things I would need to take into hospital and the members gave me some ideas. This was really useful.

Whilst the hospital provided me with a list of things I would need, this is written by someone who has not necessarily been through Chiari surgery and I found the tips from those who have, to be massively helpful. Anything to make my stay easier and more comfortable. The list I compiled is shared in the Appendix.

This activity provided me with a great distraction in the weeks before my operation. One of the items my group recommended were pyjamas that fasten at the front with buttons, rather than ones you pull over your head. These turned out to be very difficult to find in the summer. Not only that, but I also have *Koumpounophobia* which is a fear of buttons. I know, right?!

I wasn't too good on my feet at this point so actually going to a shop wasn't an option for me. Instead, I trawled the internet in search of the perfect pair. This soon changed to just any pair, and being in-between sizes at the time, I had to order two of each and hope one would fit.

I became great friends with the postman as parcels of pyjamas began to arrive every couple of days. Some I discarded straight away if the buttons were too big. Others I tried on, but they didn't fit. Or they were too short. Or too thick. The pile of discarded pyjamas grew as they waited for Andrew to take them back to the Post Office to be returned.

It became a standing joke between us and was soon known as 'pyjama gate'. Every evening Andrew would come home from work and ask how many pairs I was returning that day. Silly perhaps, but it was something we could both focus on and helped us to get through.

Eventually I found a couple of suitable styles and ordered two pairs of each. With four pairs of pyjamas, I was finally sorted…except I was kept in a hospital gown for most of my stay.

They came in useful for the next time instead.

Mid May 2018

It was time for my pre-operative assessment at the neurocentre, where I met the specialist nurse the consultant had mentioned at my first appointment.

She took some blood, checked my reflexes, and gave me a general once over to make sure I was healthy enough to have the operation. The nurse then took a comprehensive medical history from me along with a list of the medication I was on. Then she began to talk about the operation.

It was at about this point I noticed Andrew looking decidedly green. He's never been very good with medical things and so found himself whisked off to another room for a lie down and a drink of water. I think he just wanted some of the attention too!

It was my brain being operated on, but he was the one feeling sick. Bless him.

Once the Andrew diversion had been sorted, the nurse turned her attention back to me and told me to expect to be in hospital for around a week to ten days. She also asked what support I would have when I got home as I would need some help to begin with.

It all sounded straightforward, and I felt like I was in good hands. I was given all the usual leaflets about anaesthesia and one specifically for Chiari with details of exercises. These I was encouraged to begin before my operation, so that they were second nature post op. I needed to make sure that my neck didn't become stiff after surgery, otherwise that could lead to further problems including headaches. And I had had enough of those!

As the date for my operation grew nearer, Andrew and I decided to go away for a night. We chose a spa day with an overnight stay. After checking in we had a bite to eat, a drink in the bar and then went for a walk around the grounds. I was tiring easily now so it wasn't long before we were back in our room. We were fortunate though, as there was a lovely patio area to our room which overlooked the river. We were able to sit and relax as we watched the narrow boats chug past.

Not only was I tiring easily but I was also struggling in crowded areas with lots of noise and activity. For this reason, we had our evening meal in the room, and I think this was the first time Andrew really appreciated how difficult eating had become for me. I was choking on my food more regularly, something he hadn't witnessed at home so much as I usually ate separately to the rest of the family.

We had also begun to sleep in separate beds at home as I was tossing and turning, finding sleep hard to come by and would wake up struggling to breathe. In the hotel we didn't have a separate room and although I had told Andrew how I sometimes found it hard to get my breath and would wake up gasping, he was still horrified to witness this. In the end it was a broken night of sleep as Andrew watched me like a hawk and woke me every so often to make sure I was okay.

Back home it took me a good couple of days to get over the break. I was completely wiped out and hurt all over.

The only thing I had to look forward to, was the time when we would be able to go away, without me suffering when we got home.

That, however, felt like a long way away.

**

***

The Operations

***

Joanne

First Operation - June 2018

I say 'first operation' but at the time I had no idea it would be the first. I thought the surgery was going to be the answer, the solution, and whilst I understood the limits to what it could achieve, I never expected there to be two more surgeries. That was most definitely not part of the plan.

I don't remember the first operation itself – obviously. I was medicated, drugged, and anaesthetised to the point where I woke up on the main ward with no idea where I was or what time it was. The only way I got my bearings was through the staff shift changes. I woke and slept fitfully, an endless cycle of fuzziness and agony. I had no idea when or if painkillers were due, I just screamed when I needed them.

Andrew tells me I went back to ITU soon after the operation. I can only imagine how difficult that must have been for him. Those days are still a blur, but I remember telling the nurses and doctors that I didn't feel right, and they kept reassuring me that it was to be expected.

Back on the main ward I was incredibly weak, and I soon became de-sensitised to my needs and the help I required. On one occasion I managed to get to the toilet but didn't have the strength to wipe myself afterwards. A male nurse helped then took me back to bed and I realised I was beyond caring.

Getting washed wasn't an option in the early days, so the nurses gave me bed baths. At first, I couldn't do anything to help apart from roll (with assistance) to one side and the other for the sheets to be changed. It was humiliating but I was so out of it, I just had to let the nurses do their job – and they were incredible. Nothing was too much trouble. They moved me, washed me, cleaned me without question or grumbling and gradually I was able to 'help' more.

As my strength returned, I was able to move more and so we started measuring my progress in little victories such as being able to wash my own face or put on my deodorant. Aside from the gravity of the surgery, my recovery was an intensely sobering experience and I promised myself that I would never take anything for granted again. That I would achieve something every single day, no matter how small. To this day, when I have bad spells or 'blips' as I call them, I measure my progress in small victories such as, 'yesterday I wasn't able to eat but today I've had soup'.

Some gestures of those amazing staff I will never forget. One day a nurse was bathing me, when the string that had been holding my hair back (a tie from a hospital gown) was lost. Without hesitation, the nurse took the bobble out of her own hair and gave it to me so that my hair could be tidy. I worried that she would get into trouble, but she assured me it was okay. Such a small act of kindness, but one that has stayed with me because it meant so much.

Eating was a whole other challenge. Whilst in ITU I'd been on liquid feed but on the ward, as I began to gain strength, I was assessed by the Speech and Language Therapists to check my swallowing ability and reflexes. I remember that I still had the NG tube in my throat as they gave me a pot of custard and some ice cream to try which tasted incredible!

It was a real positive that I could manage to eat these, so my food began to be balanced, some liquid and some pureed. The dieticians were amazing, explaining how important it was that I had the right amount of calories, fat, and protein for my wound to heal. The pureed meals though...those I will never forget. Essentially normal food was pureed and then formed in a mould to resemble what it had been before, so a pile of carrots or baked beans. I soon learned which meals to avoid (beef steak), and which were okay (fish pie) and, I now realise that these meals were a lifesaver.

Andrew visited and would spend hours massaging hand cream into my hands – especially my right hand. The nerve damage had restricted my movement in it, and I didn't have much feeling, so the physio and occupational therapist had given me some exercises to do. Hand massage was one. They also suggested I touch and feel different textures and try pressing down the handle of a spoon whilst it was flat on the table. I had to use each finger for this and at first I managed to press down, but had no control over releasing the handle, which meant the spoon just flicked back up at me. Eventually though this got better, and I began to work with plasticine as well making balls, flowers, and petals. Simple things that I had taken for granted and I am certain that what Andrew did during that time, played a massive part in my recovery.

When I got home my niece came to visit and brought me a cushion with a word embroidered on it. The physios suggested tracing the word using different parts of my hand across the various textures to improve the feeling and sensitivity. It was a huge help.

As I began to feel stronger in the hospital, I asked one of the healthcare workers if it would be possible to go downstairs in a wheelchair for a change of scenery. I thought perhaps Andrew could take me down to the coffee shop. The healthcare worker became very excited at the prospect of my 'date' as they labelled it and scoured the cupboard on the ward for some nice toiletries to give me a bubble bath and wash my hair. She helped me into my favourite set of pyjamas and blow dried my hair and for once, I felt human. Several of the nurses popped their heads in to see how I was getting on – I think they were almost as excited as I was.

The plan was for me to have my lunch and usual nap and then go downstairs with Andrew afterwards. Unfortunately, I was so excited that I couldn't sleep which meant that by the time Andrew arrived with the wheelchair to take me on our 'date', I was exhausted. In the end he went and fetched us takeaway latte's…but at least I looked decent, and the thought was there.

Once I was feeling up to it, I would engage in conversation with anyone. One such person was a domestic helper who was from Poland. She would tell me tales of growing up in a beautiful country and why she had come to the UK. It was fascinating and helped the long days to go just that little bit quicker. I would recommend anyone who is in hospital to get to know the domestics and HCSWs especially. They will always help you when you need it and be glad to stop for five minutes to fill you in with what is going on in the world.

As I am remembering my failed 'date' with Andrew whilst writing, I find myself indulging in a wry smile. At the time we didn't worry too much because I would soon be home.

Little did we know this would be far from my last stay in hospital and that Andrew would, in fact, have many other opportunities to take me on our 'date'.

***

Timeline
Joanne - June 2018

At this point, I'd like to share the timeline of events during the first operation and subsequent stay in hospital. I think it will be beneficial to understand what that first recovery looked like, though bear in mind this was my experience based on my condition – it will be different for everyone depending on several factors, not least of which will be the type of Chiari malformation they have.

5th June 2018 ~ Admitted for operation. **Craniocervical decompression** for Chiari Malformation. I remember stopping at the services on the way as we were early and having something to eat. Dad and Daniel (son) came with me. On the ward my Surgeon went over the operation, and I signed the consent form. I think this helped Dad and Daniel too. Dad said he felt confident I was in safe hands.

> **Craniocervical decompression:** brain surgery where extra room is created for the bottom part of the brainstem and top part of the spinal cord.

6th June 2018 ~ Decompression Day. Oddly I felt calm on waking, so I tried to stay zoned out. After my shower and putting on the requisite gown I kept the curtains closed around me, lay on the bed and relaxed. I was first down to the operating theatre. I remember thinking that the operation was to save my life and there was no point in being scared. During the operation it was noted that my right tonsil was large and swollen and stuck to my brain stem. Medical notes showed it blocking the **obex**.

They dissected it off the brain stem arachnoid and **debulked and hitched**. Free flow of **CSF** was noted at the end of the procedure.

Obex: the part of the brain where the fourth ventricle narrows to the central canal of the spinal cord.

Debulked and hitched: cut, re-sected and opened.

CSF: Cerebrospinal fluid

7th June 2018: Day 1 post op ~ I complained of headache and nausea and was told this was to be expected. We noted that I had weakness in my right hand and forearm. It also felt very numb with sporadic pins and needles in the fingers. I was having trouble swallowing but they told me to have some soup. I took some but it made me cough and so I was referred to Speech and Language Therapy (SALT). On review I had a chesty sounding cough and an intermittent wet voice. They tried me with two sips of fluid and commented that my swallowing was uncoordinated. Immediately on swallowing I was coughing up green phlegm and showing signs of **aspiration**. It was recommended that I go nil by mouth. That night as Andrew left to go home, I asked him to speak to the lady opposite me and ask her to keep an eye on me overnight. I honestly felt as if I was drowning. A nurse on the meds round overheard and told me not to be daft and not to worry - they would keep an eye on me.

Aspiration: fluid 'going down the wrong way' and entering the lungs

8th June 2018: Day 2 post op ~ Again I had severe headache and nausea. I was told to sit out of bed as this should help. SALT team reassessed me and said that my swallow was unsafe so asked for an NG (nasogastric) tube to be inserted. This was done at 3.30pm by a nurse.

I was put onto liquid food by the dieticians who decided that the feed would go in from 3pm until 11am and then have a break from 11am until 3pm. Because there was a query of silent aspiration, I was sent for a CT scan and x-rays. The x-rays confirmed I had pneumonia from aspiration.

By 10pm that evening I was in respiratory decline. I was seen by the SMART team who said I was **hypoxic** with type I respiratory failure, secondary to aspiration pneumonia with worsening oxygen levels and **bulbar dysfunction** and that I would benefit from level 2 care. The decision was taken to move me to HDU with high flow oxygen, **CPAP** support and strong antibiotics. I was taken down to HDU at 11.30pm.

I don't remember anything about the transfer, just asking them to support my head when they moved me from bed to bed as I had been sick earlier. I remember feeling as if I was in the middle of a very big room with lots of beds and machines, but my family say the room wasn't that big.

I woke up at one point and a nurse was doing something and then I realised a doctor was fiddling with my wrist. I asked what he was doing. He told me he was putting some stitches in. I was so out of it I just accepted this. I now know he was putting an **arterial line** into me.

Hypoxic: when the body is deprived of oxygen

Bulbar dysfunction: the part of the brain stem that controls swallowing

CPAP: a machine that provides oxygen via a face mask and tube

Arterial line: a thin tube placed directly into the artery for ease of access to blood pressure and for blood tests

10th June 2018: Day 4 post op ~ I was now in my own room due to side effects from the feed. I remember this day as it is the anniversary of my mum's passing and I commented to the nurse looking after me that my dad may be a bit upset when he came to visit.

I was given chest physio regularly using a device called a **'Bird'** and was also encouraged to sit out of bed for short periods to help with my lungs.

I was regularly put on a **nebuliser** that delivered salbutamol to my lungs. I found the nebuliser relaxing. I couldn't talk whilst using it so always took the opportunity to close my eyes and rest. Afterwards, my breathing was easier.

> **Bird:** mechanical ventilator part operated by the patient to improve lung function

> **Nebuliser:** machine for breathing medication in mist form, via a face mask

11th June 2018: Day 5 post op ~ I was on CPAP support every four hours along with regular chest physio. I was exhausted. It was today they began to wean me off the oxygen.

12th June 2018: Day 6 post op ~ Today I had my arterial line removed and a further SALT assessment.

14th June 2018: Day 8 post op ~ I was seen by Speech Therapy again who noted that I still had high oxygen requirements and an ineffective swallow. I couldn't swallow saliva and my voice sounded wet and gurgly. They recommended that I be continued on **NBM** with the NG tube for food and nutrition.

I was discharged from ITU onto a regular ward – a different one to the first I'd been on post op – and the staff were told to readmit me to ITU if I showed any signs of respiratory distress.

NBM: nil by mouth i.e., no food or drink via mouth

16th June 2018: Day 10 post op ~ Today I have made progress. I have been able to sit out of bed for a bit longer and the **SMART** team have told me they no longer need to review me. Yay!

SMART: A team of specialist nurses who are called upon if there are additional issues/challenges for a patient.

17th June 2018: Day 11 post op ~ Today was 'sleep day' which basically means you sleep all day. Normally this happens on the second or third day after surgery, but my timings were all to pot due to having been in ITU.

My Brother came from Northumberland to see me. I think I opened my eyes for about five minutes to say hello and that was it. Andrew told me later that my dad, brother, and he had been sat by my bed for an hour or more waiting for me to wake up.

Eventually the nurse suggested they may as well go home as this was my 'sleep day' and I would be unlikely to awake. They decided to go for a coffee and give it some time but on their return I was still asleep, so they called it a day.

'Sleep day' was a blessing. I remember very little pain that day.

18th June 2018: Day 11 post op ~ My stitches were taken out today by the specialist nurses. I was also moved to a side ward because of the effect of the liquid feed on my digestive system. Not pleasant. They wanted everyone to be safe so isolated me and took cultures. The room was incredibly warm and we were in the middle of a heatwave. The sun poured in most of the day; it was stifling. Luckily the Estates Manager walked past my room and noticed the problem. He went and found some window blinds and then came back and installed them himself. They were a bit short, but I remember us laughing about it. The blinds kept some of the sun out which helped a lot. Another small gesture of kindness that I will never forget.

19th June 2018: Day 12 post op ~ I had a review with the speech and language specialist today who recommended I try sips of plain water to see how I got on. This felt like a crucial milestone.

20th June 2018: Day 13 post op ~ Another speech and language assessment today checking my swallowing ability and reflexes. I still had the NG tube down, but I was given a pot of custard to try and some ice-cream – it tasted so good!!

They were happy that I could manage these and so I was able to have these along with my feed through my NG tube. And a cup of tea. That first cup of tea was amazing! The plan was to slowly wean me off the NG feed so that I would have an appetite to increase my intake of category C / soft liquid food (custard, ice cream etc). My rest from the NG feed was now increased from 6am to 8pm. Having more rest from this made it much easier to move from the chair to the bed during the day. It felt like freedom.

22nd June 2018: Day 15 post op ~ It was noted that I was beginning to mobilise a bit better today. Dad and Andrew helped me to move around the room and to the toilet and back.

In the early days of my stay the physios had given me a **Zimmer** frame to try but I'd needed two physios to help me with this. With dad and

Andrew supporting me I felt a lot better and more mobile.

It was another incredibly hot day and the ward manager came round with ice lollies that she had bought for us all. What a lovely thought and very welcome indeed.

Zimmer frame: wheeled walking frame that can be used by patients to support their weight during walking and movement

25th June 2018: Day 18 post op ~ A bit of an incident with a Weetabix. The kitchen said they had no ReadyBrek (my usual soft porridge like breakfast) as apparently the nurses made it and not the kitchen. Without my normal alternative, they suggested I try Weetabix which was also classed a category C / soft. I tried but it got stuck in my throat and I choked. My throat felt very irritated for the rest of the day – almost as if something was stuck. One of the HCSW suggested gargling a fizzy drink and so Andrew got me some cola from the shop. This did help a little so is a tip worth remembering.

26th June 2018: Day 19 post op ~ Today the NG tube was taken out as it was beginning to irritate internally. They tried to fit one through my other nostril, but it just wouldn't go in. After a discussion with the team, it was decided we would see how I got on without the NG tube but, if I didn't take in enough food and fluid, it would have to go back in. The physio also came to see me today and suggested I go for a walk down the ward. Andrew and dad had just left me to go and watch the football in the day room and so you can imagine their surprise when I slowly shuffled past on the arm of a physio. They had to wait till I walked past the other way to make sure it was me! I waved at them, but this caused me to overbalance and stumble into the wall. I also discovered that I couldn't walk and talk at the same time which was a very strange experience.

27th June 2018: Day 20 post op ~ Today was a difficult day. I was moved back onto the main ward which was very busy and noisy. A bit of a shock after being in ITU and then my own room. I felt very low and disheartened. The lady opposite me had her mum to visit and I watched as her mum sat and brushed the lady's hair. It was a punch to the gut as I realised just how much I missed my mum. The lads were all being fantastic but sometimes you just need your mum.

I wanted to go home. I'd been in hospital for almost three weeks now and felt that I'd hit a stalemate. I wanted my own bed. My own comforts.

I had to do a stairs test with the physio to make sure I could manage going up and down the stairs. It felt irrelevant as I was planning to stay with dad in his bungalow for a few days, but it was a box that needed to be ticked. Luckily, I managed to do this.

Dad came to collect me and take me home, but we had to wait for my medications from the pharmacy. I was so glad I had ordered my tea as I was still there! A while later a nurse came to see me and knelt by the bed. I knew it was bad news. She explained that the medicines had not arrived from the pharmacy as there was a query on one of the items that needed a doctor to resolve. I asked if I could go home. They said I should stay.

I dug my heels in and argued that the consultant had said I could go home and that the physios were happy with me. I asked if someone could collect the meds the following day. Also, as I had been on most of the same meds pre and post op, I had enough to tide me over.

Eventually the medical team agreed, and I was allowed home. It had been a very, very long day.

***

***

Post First Operation

and

Second Procedure

***

Joanne
July 2018

After my first op, because I didn't have the boys at home and Andrew was working long days, we decided it would be best for me to go and stay at dads for a while.

This helped so much. Not only does he live in a bungalow so no stairs (!), but it also meant I had company and someone to keep an eye on me. In the early days you're not supposed to lift anything – including the kettle! – but fortunately Dad likes his coffee as much as I do so hot drinks were in regular supply.

Post operation I was keen to recover and get back to as normal a life as I could. This meant I would need ongoing support and appointments, but I was fine with that, if I kept going in the right direction.

These are the days after my return home. The outcome of which, I was wholly unprepared for.

18th July 2018 ~ Today I was seen in outpatients by the specialist nurses. My wound was healing well, and they were happy with that, but I was still having a lot of dizziness and needed a stick for mobilising. I was also very tired but as it was early days, I was told to be patient - which has never been one of my strong points.

The nausea had not subsided either, so I was still taking the anti-sickness tablets. Not only that, but my right hand was still giving me a lot of problems due to its weakness. They decided to refer me to occupational therapy who would assess me at my home, ready for when I moved back from dad's.

August 2018 ~ I saw my consultant in his clinic today and he told me that my Chiari had been a particularly bad one. In fact, one of the worst he'd seen in his career. I didn't know whether to be pleased at my uniqueness or terrified at its severity.

The consultant said that when they opened me up my tonsils had almost 'jumped out' because they were under so much pressure.

I told him I was still experiencing dizziness and he suggested going to the **ENT** specialists to see if they could offer any help with this part of my recovery.

ENT: ear, nose and throat specialist

28th September 2018 ~ I realised that my dizziness and nausea were getting worse and that the pains in my head were back. If I lay on my side I had the now familiar feeling of my head sinking into the pillow, as if I've had a good night out but without all the fun. I contacted my GP who spoke to the neurocentre but the system wouldn't allow my GP to refer directly, so I had to go to my local hospital first. This meant going through the whole saga again whilst the doctors decided what to do.

Unfortunately, I had been put on a trolley in the main A&E corridor whilst I was waiting where the lights were very bright. There were also lots of machines bleeping and making noises which was causing me a huge amount of stress.

Andrew kept asking if I could be moved somewhere quieter and eventually, they took me to a bay, but I was then left pretty much alone, hooked up to fluids via a drip until Andrew returned at 7am the next day.

Finally, mid-morning, a doctor came to see me and explained that I was being moved to the neurocentre so that the team there could assess me. I would have to go by ambulance to be safe. My dad came with me, and I remember it feeling a very long trip, lying down on a stretcher in the back of the ambulance. The crew were fantastic though and did everything they could to make me comfortable.

29th September 2018 ~ Once at the centre I was admitted onto a ward and the IV fluids were continued. I was seen by the SMART team and then referred to the medical team.

After twenty-four hours of being monitored I was sent for an MRI scan which showed that the Chiari had slipped. I was having a lot of pain and dizziness on turning my head, lying flat and sitting/standing. The registrar came to see me and asked if I still had the head pain and was it bad when I coughed?

I remember saying I didn't know as I hadn't coughed, so he made me do it. Oh my goodness! Yes, it hurt.

He told me the results of the MRI and that he would discuss my case with the Consultant. A decision was subsequently made to insert an **ICP** monitor to measure the pressure in my head. This was fitted in on the 3rd of October 2018 under general anaesthetic.

ICP monitor: intracranial pressure monitor (the pressure in your brain)

4th October 2018 ~ Second operation ~ I was by now having a particularly horrid symptom. When I lay down it felt as if my head was falling or sinking. Like when you've had one too many.

Whilst the ICP was in situ I was told to keep a diary of when I had any symptoms or if I was doing anything like sitting up so that this could be compared with the readings to identify any problem areas.

6th October 2018 ~ The ICP 'bolt' has been removed whilst I was on the ward. It didn't hurt at all. I felt a slight pressure and pulling, but that was it. The worst part was the stitches to the wound which stung a little! One of the doctors let me grip his hand whilst these were put in, for which I was very grateful.

I was kept in for a further couple of days observation.

8th October 2018 ~ The consultant came to see me and explained that the readings from the ICP monitor were within normal limits. He thought that a 're-do compression' was therefore the way forward. The chat was brief, but he said that I would see him in the clinic tomorrow and he would explain more.

9th October 2018 ~ I was taken down in a wheelchair to see my consultant in the clinic. He explained that the Chiari had slipped. The **tonsillar** had moved causing plugging of the original decompression and obstruction of the flow of the CSF. I was, he said, being offered a 're-do compression'.

He explained that he and another neurosurgeon would do the operation which is normal practice with a re-do. The procedure involves opening the **dura**, taking some more skull and consider inserting a plate to stop it slipping again. I felt numb but oddly relieved that they could do something. But more brain surgery?

I was scared and suddenly it occurred to me that I was being selfish. I wanted to be better than I was, to have a better quality of life yet it would put added stress on my family when there was no guarantee the re-do would actually help.

The consultant disagreed. He told me that I was brave and resilient and far from selfish, but that didn't really help. I was torn as to what I should do.

I confided in the Chiari nurse back on the ward. I told her that I was quite happy just sitting on the sofa at home with Andrew and that I felt selfish putting everyone through another operation. Forget how scared I was!

The nurse explained that sometimes the first operation doesn't always work. In my case the surgeon had been cautious as to how much bone he had removed (on the basis you can't really put it back), so he'd taken less than was perhaps needed.

I discussed my fears about ending up in ITU again with the surgeon. I couldn't bear to go through that whole experience for another operation which had no guarantees. Apparently, the procedure had been changed since my first operation and patients were now kept nil by mouth after the operation until the swallow had been established. He did however say that they would insert an NG tube during the second operation so that they could make sure all was well. They were certain I would have a much better outcome this time.

Tonsillar: your tonsils

Dura: membrane of dense connective tissue surrounding the brain and spinal cord

December 2018 ~ Unfortunately, my redo operation was delayed. At first this was due to the availability of the surgeons but then the wound from the ICP monitor wouldn't heal.

When I first became concerned that the wound was not healing, I sent a picture of it by email to the specialist nurses. They agreed that it didn't look right and arranged for me to go to the neurocentre to have it checked. It wasn't long before I was having twice weekly trips to the neurocentre to have the wound redressed. All manner of solutions were tried including honey and Aquacel rope. I was also put on a course of antibiotics as the wound had become infected.

New Year 2019 ~ The wound finally healed but my symptoms had once again worsened. On top of the usual headaches, dizziness, and nausea, I was now suffering from pins and needles in both hands and arms. It was a case of waiting again now for the re-do operation date.

11th March 2019 ~ Because I had been so unsure about having the redo, the Chiari nurses had arranged for me to be seen in the joint Chiari clinic with 3 neurosurgeons. I was very nervous on the day and had some questions ready, but I needn't have worried - they could not have been nicer.

The two surgeons that were to do my op asked me some questions about how I had been and then they outlined what they would do in the procedure. The operation, they said, was clearly necessary and knowing that alone, took some of the pressure off me having to decide.

When they asked if I had any questions, I queried if I would be able to go to my son's graduation later that year. The surgeons told me it was very possible and with that assurance, I agreed to go ahead with the operation.

2nd April 2019 ~ Today was admittance day for the re-do compression procedure. On the ward the operation was explained to me again and I tried to relax but I found it so tough. The risks were outlined with such honesty it was hard to remain positive. The surgeons informed me that the re-do procedure carried risks of severe neurological injury including stroke and paralysis as well as potential speech and swallowing problems - I was terrified.

***

***

Third Operation

***

Joanne

April 2019

3rd April 2019 ~ Third operation ~ I was remarkably calm; I think because I realised how much I needed this operation and that there really was no choice. I coached myself to be calm and let the experts do their job. When the operation was over, I was taken from recovery to x-ray to check that the NG tube inserted in theatre was in the correct position. Unfortunately, it wasn't and so it had to come out. A member of SMART team had another try that evening and this time it went in perfectly.

Now I could relax in the knowledge that I wouldn't aspirate, like last time.

4th April 2019 ~ Day one post op (3) ~ I felt quite well the day after my op. A bit headachy and nauseous as to be expected, but nothing like last time.

5th April ~ Day two post op (3) ~ I spoke too soon – today was a very bad day. I felt extremely sick, had a horrendous headache and was acutely sensitive to light and noise.

The nurses kindly drew my curtains and when Andrew and dad came to visit, they simply continued to refresh the cold flannel on my forehead. A gesture that did help a little.

I was reviewed and kept a close eye on. My painkillers were changed to try and ease the headache and a lumbar puncture was considered if the headaches were to worsen.

I was told that one way to ease headaches after the operation was to be mobile, which seems ironic when your head feels like it's going to explode! – so with great reluctance I got up and walked about ten metres with the help of two physios and a zimmer frame. I was very unsteady, but they assured me I had done well.

My headache eased a little and they told me that becoming mobile was important for another reason. The catheter needed to be removed sooner rather than later to prevent any infection.

That meant I needed to be able to use the toilet.

6th April 2019 ~ Day three post op (3) ~ I felt a lot better today and managed to sit up and be quite chatty with the doctors when they came around. The decision was taken for the catheter to be removed and they expressed satisfaction at how much progress I had made. For once it felt like something had worked.

8th April 2019 ~ Day five post op (3) ~ I was feeling very comfortable by now and we were confident that the NG tube could come out. I had been managing textured foods without any issues.

The registrar came to see me and said that in view of my excellent progress and glowing reports from all the specialists, the team had agreed I could be discharged home. We were in shock!

Andrew had taken one of the boys back to university and though my dad had turned up, he was only expecting to visit, not take me home!

My dad spoke to the nurses and told them that we had nothing ready at home and were they sure it was wise for me to be discharged? They assured him I would be fine which was so unexpected. During all the pre-operative appointments I had been told that the recovery period could be harder and longer than for the first operation and that I should expect to be in hospital for 10 – 14 days.

I didn't even have a bag or case with me to take my things home. One of the HCSW's said that I could take as many patient property bags as I needed, but I insisted that my dad go to a shop down the road and buy me a suitcase. I told him I didn't want to walk out looking like a bag lady.

9th April 2019 ~ Day six post op (3) ~ The dietician rang me at home to check how I was and to make sure I had a prescription for Ensure drinks. I said that I didn't and that I was struggling to eat and had a very low appetite.

I was also finding it hard to get up and down the stairs due to the pains in my legs and the dizziness. Andrew was at work which meant I was on my own at times and because we hadn't been expecting such a rapid discharge, we'd not made any alternative arrangements. The dietician advised Andrew to go shopping and get me lots of non-perishable snacks that I could keep in a basket in my bedroom.

She suggested high calorie drinks such as milkshakes and fizzy drinks and to try to eat and drink a little and often. She also thought my reduction in appetite was due to the adjustment, and overwhelming feeling of being back home.

My GP was contacted to get the prescription for the Ensure drinks I needed, and I got into the habit of leaving a couple in my bedroom so that I could sip them throughout the day. I also snacked on pots of custard and little packets of biscuits.

We were concerned about my mobility issues so the dietician very kindly contacted the physios to see if they could help. As I had been discharged from their care though, they advised there was nothing they could do and that I would need to speak to my GP for another referral. So frustrating.

17th April 2019 ~ Day 14 post op (3) ~ I had an outpatient appointment at the neurocentre today and the specialist nurses removed the stitches from my wound. I was still very unsteady on my feet, was experiencing pain in my coccyx and had a persistent headache. My judgement of the stairs at home was not good at all, not helped by the pain in my back. In addition, my GP had told me I had a urinary tract infection, so was on antibiotics which were making me feel groggy.

The nurse specialist advised me regarding my anti-sickness meds and told me I could change the dosage depending on my needs. This was so encouraging to hear, knowing that I had somewhere to go in terms of dosage, should I need it. I was rapidly discovering that there was nothing more exhausting than taking all my medication and still feeling unwell.

I was also advised by the team to keep up with my neck exercises which was great advice. It was and still is, so important to keep some sort of mobility and strength in my neck which can help to prevent more problems down the line including stiffness, pain, and headaches.

11th June 2019 ~ I was seen by the registrar in the outpatient's department today. He was pleased with my recovery from the redo decompression and said that the operation went well. He said I would be reviewed again in 6 months' time and have another MRI scan to check all was well.

***

JOANNE ROBERTSON

***

Life Before Chiari

***

Joanne

To give you a better insight into the effects that Chiari can have on someone's life, I thought it would be useful to tell you about my early years and how I lived pre-diagnosis. To say it changed my life irreversibly is an understatement.

I was born in the early 1970's in Oldham to the most amazing parents who met whilst working in the police force. My dad was a sergeant and, once I'd been born, mum had a variety of part-time jobs including helping at my junior school with reading lessons.

School was not my favourite place to be so as well as the reading lessons, mum often volunteered to help on school trips as she knew it was the only way she could get me to go. I had mixed emotions about mum joining these trips. On one occasion we visited the canal in Manchester and mum scolded me in front of everyone for talking to the boat driver for too long.

I had a lovely childhood though and as much as I hated school I excelled, receiving the award each year for top girl and then second in class in Juniors.

I passed all my O levels with good grades and was a keen musician, so I learned the guitar and violin. This gave me so many opportunities, not least of which was playing in the school orchestra and later appearing on television as a member of the Oldham Music Centre Youth orchestra.

I also loved to dance. I remember starting with ballet at a very young age but I was impatient. When we were doing barre exercises and pretending to be ducks and fairies, I asked the teacher when we would be doing a proper ballet, like Swan Lake. Madame was not impressed with my question and so it was that I quickly tired of ballet and what I considered to be the 'boring stuff'.

My attention shifted to Latin American dancing and ballroom which I attended for a long time and reached the highest level I could. It was a proud year when I was awarded the 'Highest Marks Trophy' in the dance school exams which coincided with the end of my compulsory education.

Due to my dislike of school I decided to go to the local college rather than stay in sixth form, plus, I still didn't know what I wanted to do career wise. In the end I chose to do a BTEC National Diploma in Business and Finance. I felt it was a safe and broad enough choice and would give me plenty of options.

College opened my eyes to lots of new friendships. I enjoyed the freedom of being further away from home, getting a bus each day and having no uniform to wear. We were treated like adults, and I loved the subjects. I also enjoyed the free periods where we could nip up the hill into town and look around the clothes shops or visit my mum at work.

I applied for lots of jobs after college. I even got through to the interview stage with an airline to become an air hostess, but I wanted a safe and secure job. So, I settled on banking.

At first the training was okay but after my first day in a branch I realised it wasn't for me. The second I got home and walked into the garden where mum and dad were, I knew how I felt was written all over my face.

"You didn't like it, did you?" asked mum. That was all she needed to say.

I stuck it out for eighteen months and things did improve. I enjoyed the counter training and talking to customers, but I didn't like the endless hours of filing statements and checking balances on a microfiche (a sheet of flat film containing data that is viewed by a specialist machine – a bit like a photo negative). The biggest drama I encountered was if the bag containing the current day's microfiche didn't arrive, I had to re-use the same one as the previous day.

I made some good friends during this time though and discovered my rock chick side. I would often go out to the pub after work on a Friday, then we would get the bus into Manchester and go to the Banshee or Rock World. I would be out until five or six in the morning, and I remember my Mum telling me that if I insisted on coming in with the milkman it would make more sense to stay at a friend's. I'm guessing she didn't appreciate me coming in at all hours.

After about eighteen months in banking, I decided to take the plunge and apply for the RAF. I was approved to be a communication systems analyst and was thrilled. Sadly, my fiancé at the time did not want to be an RAF husband and was insistent that I did not take the post.

In the end I decided to follow my parent's footsteps and apply for the police. My fiancé didn't like this decision either, so we parted ways on Valentine's Day. It wasn't that simple though.

He decided to call off the wedding but did nothing to help, which left me and my parents with the headache of cancelling all the arrangements and letting people down.

Free to make my own choice now, I continued with the application for the police force, however at the final stage interview, the force wasn't convinced I was ready. The interviewers said that as I had just come out of a long-term relationship, my decision to join the force could be a knee jerk reaction and told me to re-apply in twelve-months' time. If I still wanted to.

I felt like my world had ended at that point. Where was I to go from here?

After much soul searching, some stern words from friends and parents and a much needed 18-30's (holiday) trip to Ibiza, I decided to go back to college to study for A levels whilst waiting for the twelve months to pass.

I took Psychology, Sociology and General Studies and began a part-time job as a silver service waitress at a local venue. I also threw myself into a volunteer's role at Victim Support and Age Concern.

I loved waitressing at the functions which took place at the venue. They were long days; we did a lot of weddings which were fun but very hard work.

First, we would welcome the guests and get them seated for their silver service meal. I was proud of how proficient I got at balancing numerous plates on my arms whilst serving. After the meal was finished, the guests would move to the bar area which allowed us time to clear the tables and make the room ready for the evening reception. I loved the banter and the hustle and bustle of the day and then after work we would often go straight to a nightclub in the nearby town and party until the early hours.

Volunteering at Victim Support was a real eye opener. My job was to visit victims of crime in their homes or place of work to offer them support and help, primarily with things such as phone calls and forms. I would usually see each person a couple of times before they moved on, but there were a few who required ongoing support. I particularly enjoyed accompanying victims to court. Here I was required to sit with them and offer comfort and support before they went into the main court room. This opportunity renewed my determination to become a member of the police force.

Age Concern was slightly different in that I still offered support but, in this role, I also provided companionship. I remember going to my first lady who was called Alice. She only had one leg. The first day I went to see her she didn't answer the door so I looked through the window to see if I could locate her. She was fast asleep in her armchair which worried me for a while, until I eventually managed to rouse her.

I saw Alice at least once a week and she taught me how to play backgammon. She became an important part of my life. When she died, I asked mum to accompany me to the funeral as I thought there wouldn't be many attending.

How wrong was I? It was standing room only. I wondered where all the people had come from when they'd not seemingly been around before. But it didn't matter. I was glad to have met her and felt lucky for the times we had shared.

Eleven months after my initial application to the police I was contacted by a neighbouring force who were looking for applicants to become

Special Constables. The fact I was approached by another force made me cross and so I phoned the original force to which I had applied, stating that I had been asked to join another force as a Special Constable, yet I still wanted to be a regular. With them.

At the time I had a month left before I could 're-apply' and take the fitness test, but I told them I could not wait. In the end they agreed that I could attend the next week for the fitness test, providing I was prepared.

In the run up to that day I was full of cold – but determined. I spent all week doing sit-ups and press-ups and jogging round the block. Thank goodness we didn't have camera phones in those days – mum and dad would stand at each end of the drive with a stopwatch and make beeping sounds as they tried to replicate the infamous 'beep test'. As crazy as it sounds, it worked. I passed the fitness test and progressed through the interview stages to be appointed.

Looking back, I could appreciate that being asked to defer my application wasn't a bad thing. Even though I was still only twenty-one when I joined, that extra year had given me life skills and experiences that I wouldn't otherwise have gained. And these I knew would help when it came to my police career.

I remember, when it was time for me to leave home and go to the police training centre, dad drew me a map. I loved driving and was confident in where I was going but…my parents had decided to move to Wales whilst I was away, and dad wanted me to know how to get to their new house. This was way before sat navs and other technology.

I found joining the police daunting, but I soon settled in. We were pretty much thrown in at the deep end in fact. An instructor entered our classroom and told us that there was as riot at the local prison and that we were needed. We all thought it was some kind of test. But it wasn't. We had half an hour to get our riot gear on and arrive at the meeting point to get the bus to the prison. At the prison we were asked to form a human cordon along the entrance so that the bus loads of prisoners could be moved without incident. We were all very new and fresh faced but luckily, we did good, and the job was done.

A national paper came to visit us at the training centre and focused on the fact that so many female police officers had been called to a prison riot. They took pictures of us sitting demurely in our uniform skirts and then contrasted this with photos of us in full riot gear. The story was never published unfortunately, but I still have the photos to tell the tale.

It was whilst I was in the police that I met my husband, Andrew. He was a special constable and, though we hadn't really spoken, we were aware of each other. I had a good friend who was also a special constable and she arranged for Andrew and I to have a date on Valentine's Day. We met at a local pub, had a drink and the rest, as they say, is history.

We both knew very quickly that we wanted to be together, so we married the year after that date and welcomed our first son the year after. By the time our second son came along I knew that I couldn't continue with a career in the police. I didn't feel comfortable working in a potentially dangerous job and running the risk of the boys' growing up without me.

In those days there wasn't the option to transfer to the control room for example. The only way I could do that kind of job was if I left the force and re-applied as a civilian. Instead, I settled on a few part-time jobs whilst the boys were small and then eventually, we took the opportunity to move to Wales and be closer to my parents.

Whilst pregnant with the boys and as they were growing up, I was fortunate. I had very few health concerns and never gave it much thought. Little did I know how much my health was going to take over and control my life.

Never in a million years did I suspect there was something wrong with my brain.

~~~~~~

I think it's important to realise that having a Chiari malformation affects not only the person with the Chiari, but also the family and friends. I am very fortunate to have a loving family and some close friends who have been there for me every step of the way, but it was not without its challenges.

Before I was diagnosed there was many a time when plans would be altered at incredibly short notice due to me being ill. Sometimes it would be that I couldn't physically get ready to go out or I would be in the middle of doing my hair and would collapse onto the bed with the most horrendous pressure pain in my head and neck.

And my friends and family had to learn to understand and accept this, even without a diagnosis. My family especially became very flexible and understanding. If, for example, I had to be out of the house for work by 8.15am, then they knew I needed to be dressed and ready by 7.30am with the remaining 45 minutes allowance for relaxing. This routine gave me the best possible chance to get out of the door.

Once, I was due to meet a friend, and dad was coming with me. When he arrived at my house to pick me up, I was still getting ready, and the pressure in my head, neck, and shoulders was building. We were going to an event which meant there wasn't time to wait for me to feel better, so I had to just push through. I told Andrew and dad to get me in the car and I could rest there. Somehow, they got me ready and into the car, but we'd only driven a hundred yards up the road when I knew it was no use.

The pain and pressure were increasing and there was no let-up in sight. Dad had to go all the way round the roundabout at the end of the road and take me home.

I hated times like this. I felt like I was letting everyone down.

Chiari affects so much more than the person with the illness, and it can be hard for those around you to understand and support you, especially when their plans, hopes and possibly dreams, are constantly being changed and modified.

Everyone affected needs support. Not just the patient.

***

***

Normality?

~~~~

Tales of Life with Chiari

***

Joanne

In July 2018 and following my first operation, a close relative passed away. I could not go to the hospital to say my goodbyes as I was still too weak and open to infection. For the funeral we hired a wheelchair because I couldn't walk any distance and was very unsteady on my feet. We had to be careful that people did not hug me, and mindful of me looking up at people from the wheelchair as both activities strained my neck.

As we went into the chapel the undertaker pointed to the front of the seating because I was in the wheelchair. This meant I was 'parked up' directly facing the casket which was not at all pleasant. By the end of the service I was exhausted and knew I wouldn't be able to make it to the wake. I'd also found out that the restaurant where the wake was to be held was upstairs, so trying to get there would have been a challenge in itself. In the end we went home.

This was so not normal.

~~~~~~

After my first operation we didn't want to go abroad for our summer holiday. I still wasn't too good on my feet and got tired very quickly, so we opted for a stay in the UK. We chose a lovely lodge with a hot tub. From the bedroom upstairs I could sit on the bed and look out over a golf course to the hills and watch the sunset. It was so tranquil.

There was one bedroom downstairs which we had planned for me to use but unfortunately it had twin single beds which, when I tried them were very narrow. Not only that, whenever I turned over my vertigo kicked off and that was hugely unsettling. In the end I had one of the rooms on the first floor and dealt with the stairs as I needed to.

We took it day by day and didn't plan as we just didn't know how I would be. I remember one day we decided to go to a nearby lavender farm as I had been told that lavender is very good for vertigo. Whilst Andrew went to get us some lunch from a nearby bakery, I started to get myself ready for the trip but, by the time he got back I was absolutely exhausted. Andrew helped me up to bed, gave me my lunch and made me a cup of tea. Then I rested.

A couple of hours later I felt stronger and so we decided to try the lavender farm after all. By the time we got there most people had left which meant it was relatively quiet. We were able to sit in peace in the tearoom whilst we ate beautiful lavender scones and then afterwards, we went outside and took in the view of the rolling lavender fields. It was quiet. There was little to no noise.

I bought a couple of things from the gift shop including a lavender temple roll on which I apply to my wrists and temples when I feel dizzy or nauseous. It seems to help.

On the one hand we had a lovely day but on the other, this was...

...so not normal.

~~~~~~

One of my sons wanted some bits and pieces for going back to university so we thought it would be nice to go to Cheshire Oaks to shop and have some lunch. I was incredibly unstable on my feet and had barely any stamina, so we took the wheelchair. It was an awful experience. Many of the pavements were rough and uneven which led to a very bumpy ride.

In the shoe shop Andrew had to 'park' me up and then go off with our son to look at different shoes and trainers. Wherever he 'parked' me I seemed to be in the way of someone. It was humiliating, embarrassing and I hated feeling so completely helpless.

Later, as we were walking past a jewellery shop, I asked Andrew to take me in. It was pointless. I couldn't see high enough to look at any of the shelves. The two members of staff in the shop showed little interest in helping me and simply turned back to their conversation. I tried to get their attention and tell them that I couldn't see anything, and could they help? They ignored me. All I wanted was for one of them to bring something to me so that I could see it. There were no other customers in the shop. It wouldn't have been too much trouble. Clearly it was. I felt small, insignificant, and stupid.

The doorways to shops were another issue. Some of them were barely wide enough for the wheelchair so I had to make sure I didn't get my hand caught as we passed through or that I didn't bang my head on any shelves that were the wrong height. It had been a disaster.

Keen to make the best of a bad situation we went to the pizza restaurant. The only place they could seat us with the wheelchair was right next to the toilets. Not only was it thus the busiest part of the restaurant, it was also deeply unpleasant.

An awful day.

This was so not normal.

~~~~~~

In December 2018 we went to collect my son from university to bring him home for Christmas. Someone (aka Me!) decided it would be a good idea to visit the Christmas markets but for ease, I would be in my wheelchair.

It was horrific. I swear Andrew used me as some sort of battering ram to move people out of the way and the wheelchair felt like it was going to fall apart as we bumped over the cobbled streets. I lost count of the number of people we banged into.

Others didn't appear to see me either. When they turned around, they were looking at eye height, not expecting to see someone in a wheelchair.

Suffice to say it was not a pleasant experience and one I would not like to repeat.

This was so not normal.

~~~~~~

When I was in hospital in September 2018, a friend told me that Take That were on tour the next year. I checked the internet and saw they were due to play Anfield on the 6th of June. I thought this would be amazing for several reasons:

1. It would be the 1-year anniversary of my decompression and would be a great way to mark that.

2. It was a goal to aim for in my recovery.

3. Andrew is a lifelong Liverpool football supporter so I knew he would be pleased to be able to go to Anfield.

I used to know one of the members of Take That through work and had always joked that I would never pay a ridiculous amount to go and see him perform – but this seemed the right opportunity. I had also heard how amazing their last tour had been.

I still remember the day he left his job and told us he was going to join a boyband. We all laughed and said we'd see him back at work in six months' time. How wrong we were. He's done amazing.

So, having decided to book tickets I now had the dilemma of how to do it.

The tickets were due to go on sale the next morning at precisely the same time the doctors would be doing their ward round. I knew the tickets would sell out fast so decided to take myself off to the toilet and join the booking queue whilst hoping I didn't miss the doctors.

I finally got to the front of the queue and selected tickets which faced the stage so I wouldn't have to twist my neck. All was going well until… it asked me to sign into my booking account. I didn't have one!

Suddenly I remembered that my son had an account, so frantically I called him to get the tickets for me. He managed it. I couldn't believe my luck.

It was with some relief and a huge smile therefore, that I made it back to bed just in time for the doctor.

One of the nurses asked why I was grinning from ear to ear, and I told her. I was so excited about the prospect of having something on the calendar to look forward to.

The date drew nearer – and sadly I realised I would not physically be well enough to go. The trip to Liverpool alone would wipe me out, never mind sitting through a concert and all the noise that would entail. Reluctantly, we sold the tickets to a friend. I believe they had a great time so at least someone got to enjoy it.

This was so not normal.

~~~~~~~

For Andrew's Birthday I booked us tickets to go and see War of The Worlds in Concert in Leeds. We had picked Leeds so that my son, who was at university nearby, could come along too.

This turned out to be yet another trip I couldn't attend. The boy's told me after the event that there was no way I could have gone. The seats had been high up which would have caused me problems with vertigo, not to mention the volume at which the orchestra played.

It was incredible, they said, but too much for me.

This was so not normal.

~~~~~~~

When the boys left home to go to university, this was meant to be our time – mine and Andrew's. Never did we consider that Andrew would become my carer.

I was able to help both the boys move into the accommodation for their first year but after that it was all up to Andrew. I really feel that I missed out on so much.

After my first operation I did make the odd trip to see them, but it proved to be expensive as we would need to break the journey with an overnight stop. We'd also then have to stay another night before heading back home.

The pressure on dad and Andrew to do all the driving was too much, whereas before we would have shared the driving between us.

This was so not normal.

~~~~~~

.

***

Long Lasting Effects

***

Joanne

And now we reach the point where there is little else to my story save for the long-lasting effects that Chiari and three brain surgeries have left me with. Some are good, some not so good and you may experience all or none of these. They are simply facts of where I am now.

Dignity

During my time in hospital I lost all sense of dignity. At first I was too ill to care, but as I recovered, I became aware of what was going on and felt acute embarrassment. Like everything else with Chiari though, this was perfectly normal and now I understand that dignity is something I have relinquished when it comes to my health.

Strength

If I feel strong enough to walk the dogs then I must go with at least one other person, but often there are two with me. I can't hold the leads firmly as my grip strength is poor and the dogs can easily pull me off balance. Sometimes the leads will get tangled around my feet and that can be very challenging to negotiate.

Our preference these days is to go to the beach where I can sit on the wall and watch as Andrew walks the dogs.

When one of our dogs became elderly, we bought her a doggy pram, which was great for me too. I could push the pram and use it for balance. Sadly, she is no longer with us. I suppose I could push an empty pram around but that would probably result in me getting some very strange looks.

Emotions

After the last of my three surgeries, I found that my emotions were all over the place. I would break down in tears at the weirdest things and sob uncontrollably. This took almost a year to overcome. Though some of it was undoubtedly due to the surgery, I am sure that much was a result of being physically and mentally spent. To this day, my emotions can still be all over the place, especially when I am overtired or stressed.

Friends

This is something I wasn't expecting. Sadly, I have lost many friends over the years. Pre-diagnosis I was erratic and prone to letting people down which some were unable to understand. And I get that. I had hoped that once I'd received my diagnosis and there were reasons for my behaviour, friends I lost would get back in touch but unfortunately that hasn't happened.

There are some friends though who have stayed with me throughout and been absolutely amazing. In the *Hints and Tips* section there are some suggestions of things my friends have done for me which really helped. Hopefully you will have some special people who can do those things for you too.

Decisions

If I have too many options I find it incredibly tough to make a decision. If I'm asked what I want to eat, half the time I have no idea. We find it easier for Andrew to decide most things, particularly when it comes to where we need to go as a family. I simply have to be told when and where, and I'll be ready.

I appreciate this is not ideal and puts (further) pressure on Andrew but if I am given too many choices, I become overwhelmed and confused which leads to stress and an exacerbation of my symptoms, so we may end up going nowhere.

The only downside is I don't get to complain if we go somewhere I don't like!

Car Journeys

I have to rest my head on a cushion during car journeys to reduce the feeling of the vibrations. In fact, I always take plenty of cushions with me in the car. I often need to rest my right arm too because this becomes heavy with pins and needles after a while. I also change the seat settings often to make sure I can find the most comfortable position.

Conversations

I find conversation challenging as I often lose my train of thought and struggle to find the right words to say. I also find it exhausting to talk and even nodding my head in agreement can quickly exacerbate symptoms.

Environment

I am completely unable to function in noisy or busy environments. They are just simply far too overwhelming.

Confidence

I have none. It's all gone. It's that simple.

Tolerance

On a bad day, that's also gone. The level is zero.

Personal Care

I have raisers fitted to my toilet to help with my balance. I would definitely recommend taking advice from an Occupational Therapist as they can provide all manner of equipment to help. I also have a shower stool, perch stool for the kitchen and a walker.

I am unable to have a bath. I don't have the strength to get in and out of the bathtub. I'm okay with showering but find it incredibly tiring so we've now got a routine in place that kind of works. Andrew will make me a cup of tea whilst I shower then I will sit on the bed with my feet up whilst I drink my tea and recover some energy.

If it's a hair wash day, then I will wrap my hair in a towel and relax for a while until I have the energy to brush it through. I find that it helps to do this in stages.

If I did it all in one go then it would wipe me out for the rest of the day.

Planning

I cannot plan long term as I have no idea how I will be from one day to the next. I can wake up fine but then after doing something, be absolutely floored and out of action for the rest of the day. I find it impossible to work to a deadline or tight schedule for that exact reason.

The days when I knew what was coming next are long gone.

***

Making Chiari make sense ~ for others

***

The Spoon Theory

It can be really hard to make someone understand how your energy can be up and down so much and how you can do something one day and not another.

The fact that Chiari is an invisible illness makes it even harder. I like to refer to "The Spoon Theory", which is a personal story by Christine Miserandino. It is popular among many people dealing with chronic illness and is used to describe the amount of mental or physical energy a person has available for daily activities and tasks using "spoons" as a unit of energy.

Christine Miserandino lives with lupus and one day her best friend asked her what it was like to live with a chronic illness. They were in a café at the time so Christine grabbed the nearest things - spoons - and used them to represent units of energy. She explained that when living with a chronic illness energy is limited and depends on many factors such as stress, how we're sleeping, and pain.

Christine then went through her friend's day taking spoons, or energy, away from the friend as she listed the things she did.

The friend soon realised that it didn't take long for her to run out of spoons, meaning she functioned for a good part of the day on empty.

With Christine though and her chronic illness, she automatically started the day with less spoons and would need to use up more spoons to carry out simple tasks. Thus, her spoons (or energy) would deplete significantly faster and could take longer to refill.

Many people find it useful to use this 'spoon' theory to explain to friends and family that they just don't have it in them to cook the tea, meet for a coffee or do the housework that day.

When suffering with a hidden illness there can be feelings of guilt that you are letting family and friends down or that you can't contribute as much as you would like. The spoons theory is a good way to illustrate and help someone visualise your daily struggle and what you want to do versus what you can do.

In time you will become adept at allocating your spoons to what works best for you. For example, it might use three spoons to collect your children which might prevent you from meeting up with a friend. If there is a day when you don't collect the children though, you could use these three spoons for your friend.

If you plan how you are going to spend your spoons, then it can be a great way to manage not only your own expectations but those of your family and friends.

How you use your spoons is up to you and over time it will become second nature.

***

Working with Chiari

***

Working with Chiari

Having always been active and someone who wanted to work, I found it incredibly challenging when my illness began to affect my working life.

At the time of my diagnosis and first surgery I was working for the NHS as a switchboard supervisor, and I used to find the noise levels from the main room unbearable. If I needed to concentrate, I found the only way I could manage was by closing the door to my office which was not always appreciated by my colleagues. Sometimes the other staff felt I was shutting them out which could not have been further from the truth. There was no malice in what I did, it was simply that my brain couldn't cope with the sensory overload from all the different noises.

My balance, as with my everyday life, was also an issue. There would be times when I was walking around the office and if I turned my head or looked up or down, I would need to hold onto the wall to steady myself. Otherwise, I would have fallen.

The pain in my head became so severe that I had to support it with my hand. It felt as though my head weighed a ton and was about to explode, which made even the simplest of tasks difficult.

I remember once being so busy and short staffed that instead of working in the back office, I was asked to take calls on the switchboard. I watched the calls build up and up but was unable to move my head, to the point where my colleague checked on my welfare. I could barely speak above a whisper to answer.

As I was recovering from my first operation and preparing for my re-do, it became clear that a return to the work life I knew, was not going to be possible. I took advice from my specialist who was in no doubt that I would not be able to return to full time employment or indeed any regular employment. My balance was all over the place, I was struggling with movement of my right hand and arm, my walking distance was severely limited and that's before I'd even considered my inability to concentrate or function in a workplace environment.

It was shattering to hear it said though. I had worked all my adult life and especially in my last career I'd worked hard to climb up the organisational ladder, and to build a solid and dependable reputation. People knew me and knew that I would deliver on any task I was given, so to be told that this had been taken away from me felt so cruel.

I felt like my work life defined who I was and what I stood for and now I had nothing to anchor myself to. Or so I thought.

By necessity I have re-evaluated my life and realised the only things that really matter are your family, friendships, and your health. For so long I had put work ahead of my health and in some cases my family.

Before my diagnosis I had literally been at the stage where I would wake up early after a broken night sleep to take painkillers. I took them early enough so that they would have time to work, and I could then attempt to get out of bed. I would then get ready in fits and starts depending

CHIARI AND ME - IT'S NOT JUST A HEADACHE

on how much the pain in my head and body would allow. Often, I would have a shower then support my head by lying on the bed whilst I waited for the head pain to pass. Then I would do my hair, rest again and so it continued. It was a slow and laborious process.

Somehow, I would get through the workday but when I got home, I'd often go straight to bed. I hardly saw Andrew and I am eternally grateful of his unwavering support, when we had no idea what was wrong with me or how long it would last.

Whilst I was off sick, I was having appointments with the Occupational Health Department. Some of these were over the phone which in theory were supposed to be easier – but they were not. In many ways it was harder.

Anyone with Chiari will tell you that sometimes it hurts to even speak, which I know sounds incredible, but it really does. If, as Chiari sufferers, we could simply mumble our way through life and talk in one syllable words with no change in pitch, we might be able to struggle through, however humans don't speak or communicate this way. We must raise our voices to be heard, alter our pitch to reflect and emphasise certain emotions, and move our heads in conversation. Do you have any idea how many times we move our heads in a typical conversation?

It is thought that 55% of the meaning of a conversation is generated by our face and body, and another 38% is derived from the way we speak, e.g., our tone, volume, pitch etc. For someone unable to move their head or change the cadence of their voice due to extreme pain, it can be incredibly difficult to entertain even the shortest of dialogues. I found it then (and still do), hard to explain my condition and to illustrate how it affects me on a daily basis. Even now, when I'm in the midst of a flare up, having a conversation with Andrew can be so challenging.

It's difficult for him to understand me when I can't nod my head in agreement or utter any words.

Which is yet another reason for writing this book.

To educate.

To try to explain.

To give voice and support to those who have no hope of understanding our lives.

On the days when I had face to face meetings with Occupational Health, it took a huge effort to even get me out of the door.

I was in a wheelchair at this point so not only was the transition from house to car a challenge in itself, navigating parking spaces and kerbs at the hospital was a whole other level.

To make it worse, I was in the room literally five minutes. The Occupational Health doctor looked at me and said although it was clear at this point that I would not be able to return to my job, we couldn't come to any sort of decision that day. He said, because I was due to have my decompression operation in a couple of weeks, I would need to be reviewed after that.

It is a common preconception that decompression surgery for Chiari solves everything, and it simply does not. There is no cure. The operation merely hopes to pause a person's symptoms at that point in their lives and anything else is a bonus. There are no guarantees.

After my re-do decompression, the Occupational Health Department and HR consulted with my specialist and confirmed that they were unable to offer me any suitable amendments to my job role or office environment. My neurosurgeon further agreed that the effects of my condition and the surgeries I had undergone would make it impossible for me to hold down a full-time job.

My mobility and dexterity were severely compromised, and I was unable to concentrate for any significant length of time, so I knew what they were saying was the only outcome. That didn't make it any easier to hear or come to terms with though.

One thing I had been told by my HR department was that at the point I submitted an ill health application, my contract would be terminated. I knew this was something I had to do but my anxiety was through the roof. I felt incredibly vulnerable and worried about my wages and money not coming in – would we be able to pay the bills?

All this turmoil around work and money was going on during the preparation for and completion of my de-compression surgery, which meant it was a worrying and stressful time. I was having to make crucial decisions about lump sum payments, commutations etc, at a time when I was vulnerable and in a lot of pain. I tried speaking to a pension's advisor, but this proved almost impossible and there were days when it just hurt to speak. Not only that but my energy levels were on the floor.

I delegated as much as I could to Andrew, but often found that whoever I was speaking to would only deal with me and not with Andrew. We tried to get authority for him with as many providers as we could, but it was hard going. Some still insisted on speaking to me and to be honest, I didn't need the hassle. Even answering a couple of security questions would leave me wiped out and I just wanted to be left alone to recover. Or try to.

Any physical meetings I needed to attend around work, I had to take

Andrew with me. Not only to drive but also to assist me in the meeting. My physical and mental limitations were full on at that time and, it was beyond me to understand all that was said and requested. Even this wasn't simple. Company policy stated that when attending a sickness review you could have a colleague or a union representative with you - but not a family member. I had to ask for special permission to have Andrew there with me.

Crazy, but I did it.

I needed him there as my carer and my interpreter, someone to explain things to me after the event – often several times over. He was also my mouthpiece on the days when I literally could not speak. It's exhausting going over and over the same things all the time so in some ways, Andrew having this 'role' in my life helped him to understand more how I was feeling and what pressure I was under.

Regardless of what anyone tells you, don't be afraid to ask to have a family member attend meetings with you. It's the most invaluable thing they can do for you during your own Chiari journey.

***

***

Life with Chiari ~ Hints, Tips and Things You Need to Know

***

Disclaimer: I am not medically trained. Any advice I give in this section is purely learned from my own experiences and good old trial and error.

1. Booklet

I found it helpful to download a Chiari booklet which I sent to my line manager along with members of my family to help them understand a little about my condition. I also printed copies for my immediate family and kept a further copy to hand for any visitors who called. I found it much easier to show them a picture of what had happened to my brain, rather than try to explain it.

The booklet can be found at:

www.brainandspine.org.uk/our-publications/booklets/chiari-malformation

When I was first diagnosed and my young goddaughters visited me in the hospital, they asked me "where is your ouch?"

I did my best to explain in simple terms, but I don't think they really understood.

They had brought with them a gift, a box of Maltesers, one of which was misshapen with extra biscuit on the side. I used this to demonstrate by showing them what my brain was like now (the misshapen sweet), and then I bit off the extra to show them a nice round Malteser which signified a normal brain. This was not remotely scientific and I'm sure wouldn't stand up in the lecture halls of a medical school, but it seemed to satisfy their questions and curiosity.

2. Visitors

As my condition progressed, I found it hard to have visitors. Just talking left me feeling exhausted and in pain. I'm sure that this was very hard for people to understand, and I didn't wish to appear rude by taking myself off to a dark quiet room.

If anything, it was a little easier after surgery because people were conscious of not outstaying their welcome. I found that if I had a visitor and they stayed for about an hour this was enough to wipe me out for that day and indeed the day after.

My social circle has definitely shrunk – I'm guessing because friends have become weary of me cancelling plans – but unfortunately this is one of the features of having Chiari, it has no regard for your social calendar. If it wants to flare up, it will.

I guess this is more a fact than hint or tip but what I want to get across is how important it is to have visitors on your terms, especially in hospital otherwise it can really set you back.

3. Pace Yourself

Once I was diagnosed and we had a better idea of what we were dealing with, I started being a bit kinder to myself. I learnt how to pace myself. My family were a huge help with this. They began to know the signs of when things were getting too much for me, or when I had done too much, often before I did.

For example - I remember once going to a shop for something and then getting a coffee. I wanted to go to another shop, but my husband could see on my face and in my posture that I was reaching my limit.

He insisted that we start the half hour drive home, and I disagreed. However, as he helped me back into the car, I felt such a sense of relief. I had to admit I was wrong, which doesn't happen often in our marriage!

We quickly learnt that if I wanted to do something say on a Tuesday, we would need to allow me to do almost nothing for the 2-3 days before to give me the best chance of keeping that appointment on the Tuesday. We also learnt that the few days after were a write off whilst I recovered from the pain and exhaustion of that day.

4. Ideas for friends and relatives

If there are a few of you able to visit, have a chat amongst yourselves and arrange a schedule of who will visit when. Lots of hospitals and wards have limited visiting hours and numbers.

I would suggest that you speak to the main carer/visitor and coordinate with them. Perhaps you could offer to drive the main carer that day to give them a break, and you could check if they need you to take anything into the hospital such as clean nightwear, drinks, juice etc.

Wherever you visit them, try not to outstay your welcome. By the time the patient is showing signs of fatigue, that is too late, so watch for cues. Maybe set out an expectation at the beginning to save the patient worrying. Tell them it's only a flying visit, for example, and that you will stay for half an hour, but they must tell if you if they're tired before then.

When you are recovering from Chiari surgery or indeed most days with Chiari, every little thing you do takes that much more effort and so the patient will tire very quickly. Just the act of talking and raising their voice to be heard can be exhausting. Maybe sit and have a cuppa with them and tell them a bit of gossip so that they aren't doing all the talking. Also ask if there is anything you can do - like load the dishwasher or take the dog out – and then take your leave. This way you will both be keen to repeat the experience.

5. Ideas for presents

• One of my good friends made me a box containing a colouring book, pencils, hand cream and sock slippers, all of which were useful. It was simple, but lovely.

• Another present I enjoyed was a cuddly toy and these have become my mascots. On the days when I can't face visitors and feel alone, something cuddly can really bring comfort. It's also been great for me to squish and squidge them whilst trying to get strength back in my hand.

• Notebooks and pens were great gifts, especially when I was in hospital. I could make lists so that I didn't forget to tell my family something or ask them to bring things in for me that I needed. Now that I am home, I have one by my bedside always so I can make notes (or write books!) when I can't sleep.

• Magazines are fantastic. I can't remember the last time I had the strength to hold a book or the ability to concentrate long enough to read. I much prefer magazines that I can flick through and pick up as and when. As a bonus, when you're in hospital, you can pass these around the ward for the other patients after you've finished with them.

6. Car Journeys

I take lots of cushions to support me on car journeys as I find I have to rest my head on a cushion to reduce the feelings from the vibrations. My right arm also gets heavy, so I rest this too. It's a good idea to ask the driver to plan the journey and factor in regular stops. Plan where the toilet stops are and make sure you arrive at your destination in good time.

This is so that you can rest and gather yourself before getting out of the car. You will also not need to rush around if you do this, which is an added benefit. Rushing around can cause you to become flustered and overwhelmed.

7. Holidays and day trips

These may well look a lot different than they did before your diagnosis. We had, for example, planned to go on a cruise for our 25th Wedding Anniversary however due to my unsteadiness and vertigo, we didn't feel this was such a good idea.

Do your research. Phone in advance to check access to things like restaurants and toilets. It could be the nicest café in the town but if the toilets are up a steep flight of stairs, then you may have to rethink. I have found though, that some places will let you use the disabled or even their staff toilet if you explain your situation.

Try to avoid going at busy times if noise is a trigger. You can search online to find out how busy somewhere is at particular times of the day.

8. Hugging

It sounds such a simple thing, but a hug around your neck could really trigger your symptoms. The ones from friends around your shoulders are usually okay, but if you ever have one of those awkward, round the neck, type hugs it could bring on unwelcome symptoms. It's worth educating those around you if this is the case.

9. Don't get constipated!

If you are on a lot of pain killers, then unfortunately constipation can be an unpleasant side effect. I really recommend speaking to your GP if you think this may be the case. Straining on the loo can be extremeley painful in your head (I know, sounds crazy), so it's best to avoid this if possible.

You can also try to keep as mobile as possible because this will help your bowels and internal organs to continue to function more effectively. Again, this is just something I have discovered as opposed to a medical recommendation.

10. The Internet

I don't care what anyone says, it's impossible not to use the internet for research once you have been told you have a Chiari malformation. Doctors will advise you not to do this but there were things I just had to look up and find out.

If you are going to do some research online, try to stick to official websites such as the NHS or use resources provided to you from the hospital you are being treated at.

I have put some useful contacts and websites at the back of the book.

When searching you will come across things that you don't understand. This is normal and it illustrates precisely why doctors need to study for years to even begin to comprehend our brain, how it works and all its parts. What I found the most useful was to learn and understand some of the basic terms. This made it easier for me to know what the specialists and teams were telling me, and it also made some of the processes a little less scary.

11. Ask Questions

For my first operation I didn't care, I just wanted them to fix me, and I felt like I handed my body, brain, and everything else over to the experts to do just that. However, for my second and third procedures I was more aware and armed with a bit more information. This enabled me to ask some of the right questions and feel more confident in what they were doing and what was going to happen.

It's likely that your family and friends will want to understand too, so don't be afraid to ask questions of your doctors, nurses, and specialist teams. Anything you can learn that helps you live with your Chiari is a massive bonus.

12. Dining Out

When phoning to book a restaurant or even as a walk in, don't be afraid to ask for softer seats (or firmer if you so wish) or for a quiet table, or one easily accessible to the toilets. Your server will usually be only too pleased to grant your wish. After all, if you are happy and comfortable you are more likely to stay and order dessert or an extra drink.

I think sometimes we are too polite and when asked, "is this table okay?", we will just say yes, so as not to create a fuss. There was one occasion my friend and I went for an afternoon tea and our server sat us right next to the speaker in an almost empty restaurant. I knew it would be awful for me and so we asked to move and were accommodated quickly and without fuss.

13. Rearrange your Furniture

If you're anything like me, you'll find it very uncomfortable to look upwards because it puts pressure on your neck and causes a lot of dizziness. Likewise, I am unable to bend down to get something out of a low cupboard without overbalancing so we found it best to rearrange our cupboards so that those items I might need whilst in the house on my own were at eye level and did not involve moving anything else to get to them.

My advice would be to think what you might need from the kitchen cupboards in a typical day, be it teabags, or a can of soup. It may take a bit of rearranging, but it will be worth it in the long term.

Likewise with your wardrobe and drawers, have the items that you wear most often easily accessible, even if it means leaving them on a chair in your bedroom. I have a very awkward high shelf in my wardrobe that I need to reach up to, so I no longer use that and have all my clothes easily accessible.

14. Decompression Operation

When you have this operation, you will be laid on your front so expect to feel like you have been hit by a ton of bricks when you come round. Also, remember that this surgery is not a cure, merely a way for your symptoms to be paused at the point they are at.

15. Feelings of Relief

It may sound strange, but I was always worried that the doctors would tell me that my condition was 'not that bad'. Even when I was hooked up to monitors and saw the figures going up and down, I was terrified I would still be no further forwards.

When a doctor finally looks at your scans or listens to you and agrees that there is a reason for your immense pain it is a huge sense of relief. This is a feeling that I know many Chiari patients have.

16. How common is a Chiari malformation?

According to **www.ninds.nih.gov** it was estimated that the condition occurs in approximately 1 in 1,000 births. The increased use of diagnostic imaging though has shown that in fact, this condition may be much more common.

17. Chiari as a recognised condition

Chiari is, I have found, to be a very under-recognised condition. I applied for a brain injury card which I could show when I was out and about in a shop or restaurant or a taxi so that people could understand that I was ill. On occasion, sufferers have been mistaken for drunks as they slur their speech or cannot get their words out, and this can be incredibly demeaning and frustrating. Unfortunately, my application for this card was declined because I am not deemed to have a brain 'injury', I have a brain condition.

It would be amazing if there was something similar for brain condition sufferers as our condition is usually invisible and hard for others to understand.

18. Those Annoying Comments

People mean well but I did get to the point where I wanted to allow myself to fall or collapse, just so they could see I really did have a problem. Everyone around me kept saying they had headaches too and had I tried this tablet or that tablet…to the point I would have screamed if I'd been able to.

Hopefully this book will help you to show others that you have a condition and it's not just a headache.

19. Public Profile

Since my diagnosis I have been very excited to see Chiari Malformation featured on programmes like Grey's Anatomy, and on a phone-in on This Morning. Sadly though, I felt that these didn't go far enough to explain the condition and how it affects people, leaving viewers with the idea that it is 'just a headache'.

Awareness is key and anything we can do to raise the public profile of Chiari and general awareness must be done.

***

***

Life with Chiari ~

Symptoms

***

What are the symptoms of Chiari Malformation?

Headaches are the classic sign of Chiari malformation, especially after sudden coughing, sneezing, or straining.

Other symptoms vary and may include:

• Neck pain

• Hearing or balance problems

• Muscle weakness or numbness

• Dizziness

• Difficulty swallowing or speaking

• Vomiting

• Ringing or buzzing in the ears (tinnitus)

• Curvature of the spine (scoliosis)

• Insomnia

• Depression

• Problems with hand coordination and fine motor skills

There are different types of Chiari Malformation:

Chiari Malformation Type 1

In Chiari Malformation Type 1, signs and symptoms usually appear during late childhood or adulthood. Headaches, often severe, are the classic symptom of Chiari malformation. They generally occur after sudden coughing, sneezing, or straining.

People with **Chiari Malformation Type 1** can also experience:

• Neck pain

• Unsteady gait (problems with balance)

• Poor hand coordination (fine motor skills)

• Numbness and tingling of the hands and feet

• Dizziness

• Difficulty swallowing, sometimes accompanied by gagging, choking, and vomiting

• Speech problems, such as hoarseness

Less often, people with **Chiari Malformation Type 1** may experience:

• Ringing or buzzing in the ears (tinnitus)

• Weakness

• Slow heart rhythm

• Curvature of the spine (scoliosis) related to spinal cord impairment

• "Abnormal breathing, such as central sleep apnoea, which is when a person stops breathing during sleep" (Ref: "What is complex Chiari? – Rampfesthudson.com")

Chiari Malformation Type 2

In Chiari Malformation Type 2, a greater amount of tissue extends into the spinal canal compared with Chiari Malformation Type 1.

The signs and symptoms can include those related to a form of spina bifida called myelomeningocele that nearly always accompanies **Chiari Malformation Type 2**. In myelomeningocele, the backbone and the spinal canal haven't closed properly before birth.

Signs and symptoms may include:

- Changes in breathing pattern

- Swallowing problems, such as gagging

- Quick downward eye movements

- Weakness in arms

Chiari Malformation Type 2 is usually noticed during a pregnancy ultrasound.

"It may also be diagnosed after birth or in early infancy."

(Ref: "Paediatrics' Exam 2: Spina Bifida Flashcards | Quizlet")

Chiari Malformation Type 3

In one of the most severe types of the condition, **Chiari Malformation Type 3**, a portion of the lower back part of the brain (cerebellum) or the brainstem extends through an abnormal opening in the back of the skull.

This form of Chiari Malformation is diagnosed at birth or with an ultrasound during pregnancy.

It has a higher mortality rate and may also cause neurological problems.

***

My Symptoms of Chiari Malformation and How It Affects Me

1. Pain/pressure in my head when moving my head, looking up, getting up from bending, coughing, laughing, straining on the loo, sneezing, or any loud noises.

2. A lost voice.

3. Parts of my body are extremely sensitive to pain on touching.

4. I feel like it stops me living. I hardly see my husband, I can't take the dogs for a walk, I can't bend to do anything at a low level, and I can't help dad, who I care for.

5. I have an unsteady gait and stagger when walking. I feel drunk most of the time.

6. General neck pain and a feeling of heaviness in the back of my head.

7. Overbalancing. This happens when I move my head quickly or go from sitting to standing.

8. I have reduced strength in my right leg.

9. Dizziness. This is constant whenever I walk or move my head from side to side. If I am out with family or friends, I have to sit at the end of the table so that I am only looking one way and not moving my head from side to side.

10. I find it really hard when there is a lot of noise and sounds of different pitches. Like the washing machine on a spin cycle. It causes ringing in my ears and can be unbearable.

11. My right elbow twitches.

12. My right hand and forearm are icy cold most of the time.

13. I have blurred vision.

14. I have many episodes where I go cold and clammy or feel shaky, dizzy and unwell. I have to lie down when these occur.

15. My scalp itches.

16. Nausea. I feel sick most days and if I'm not nauseous then I will have a muzzy feeling in my head.

17. My sinuses feel blocked.

18. Eating is a challenge as I can choke on anything, no matter how small or its consistency. This has led me to avoid eating with my family or in social environments.

19. Sometimes I forget how to swallow, and I have to tell myself mentally how to do this and force myself to swallow.

20. Hiccups. These can be spontaneous and will lead to severe head pain.

21. Breathing. At my worst, when I breathed in it was like my breath would hold or skip a breath cycle. I had to tell myself to breathe again.

22. Often, I would wake up gasping for air as I 'forgot' to breathe when I was asleep. This is terrifying and can still happen on occasion.

23. I am forgetful and I muddle my words. I can no longer multi-task.

24. Bright lights can aggravate the pain in my head and increase this to a severe level.

25. During my time in hospital, liquid that I drank would often run straight out of my nose.

26. I have very little control on my temperature and find it hard to moderate. I am either too hot or too cold and there doesn't seem to be a happy medium.

27. Car journeys are incredibly difficult due to the vibrations bringing on head pain and nausea.

28. I find it very hard to fall asleep which has led to insomnia. Even when I do fall asleep, I wake often.

Remember ~ you are not alone.

★★★

***

The Final Word

***

The Final Word

It seems only fitting that I leave the final word, the summary of this book to my husband who has been the most incredibly supportive partner I could ever have asked for. Whilst I know how I feel and what I have gone through, I've only been able to imagine the impact this condition has had on Andrew and my family and I am so grateful that, through the process of writing this book, I have been able to understand a little bit more about his battles – because they are very real too.

~~~~~~

Andrew

Today

After Joanne's first operation in June 2018, she went to stay at her dad's bungalow so that she would have someone with her whilst I was at work and so she wouldn't have to contend with the stairs at our house or worry about the dogs.

I would finish work and then go and check on the dogs, sometimes grab some tea and then head over to see Joanne. It was only 10 minutes away, but it felt further.

I knew it was best for her in the short term, but I just wanted her home and some normality back in her life. I would stay for an hour or two and then she would be ready for bed so I would leave.

I saw her getting steadier on her feet slowly but surely, and a little bit of the old Joanne coming back. However, this was to be short lived. Joanne seemed to improve but then hit a wall. She would describe how her headaches were coming back and how when she lay down to sleep, she felt as though the room was spinning. We had been told that surgery wasn't a cure, but we seemed to be going back a step every day.

Things came to a head two months after her first operation in the September. I took her to see the GP and we again had to tell the GP of Joanne's condition, how she had had one operation and how she was feeling now. Joanne could hardly hold her head up she felt so ill, and she told me she thought her head was going to explode.

The GP was lovely and said that Joanne needed to go to accident and emergency. We insisted Joanne was not in any position to sit for hours on a chair in a busy noisy waiting room and eventually be seen by a doctor with no knowledge of Chiari. The GP told us that she was not able to refer direct to the neurocentre, just to our local hospital. But she did ring them rather than just sending us off with a letter. When I heard her say, "I have a very poorly lady here", my heart sank.

What were we facing? Had the operation failed?

Sitting in the A and E waiting room with Joanne was so frustrating, and I could see how painful it was for her. By the time we got through to triage, Joanne was as white as a sheet and in a lot of pain and discomfort. Every noise or movement was agony for her.

I asked the nurse if there was somewhere quieter for us to wait, and she managed to find a treatment room that wasn't in use.

We weren't in there long though as we were soon moved out into the busy corridor when the room was needed and subsequently 'parked' in front of the nurse's station. This meant we were surrounded by beeping machines, telephones constantly ringing and bright overhead lights.

I asked numerous times if Joanne could be moved to somewhere quieter given her condition. They simply said to be, 'careful what I wished for'.

Finally, in the early hours of the morning, Joanne was moved to a room in a side ward, far away from the nurse's station. She was given IV fluids and told that someone would be round to see her shortly. By now it was 2am and I really needed to get home and sleep as I was due in work in a few hours. I called back to see her at 7am, only to discover that no one had been to see her since I'd left. They hadn't even filled up her water jug.

Let's just say I soon found the nurse in charge to see what was going on.

Unfortunately, she could only tell me that the doctors would be round to see Joanne soon. I felt so helpless and frustrated. I wanted to help my wife, but I was powerless. This was such an awful position to be in and I had to go to work. I left my number with the nurses, just in case there were any developments.

At about 10am Joanne rang to say that a doctor had been to see her, and she was being transferred to the neurocentre. Her dad was with her now, but they'd told her she would be transferred via an ambulance, rather than a car. In case of any complications en-route. This was serious.

The next couple of days passed in a blur of waiting for news, and tests to see what was happening. When we were told that Joanne needed another operation, I was really concerned. Although in the scheme of things ICP monitoring is a relatively small operation, we could not help but compare it to the operation a couple of months earlier, when Joanne had ended up in ITU.

I had the day off work when Joanne had her second operation, and it was awful to see her so frightened as they wheeled her down for surgery. I waited anxiously by her bed, pacing, checking my watch, wishing the nurses would appear to tell me she was okay.

The first time I saw her on the trolley after the surgery, I can't describe the relief I felt. She had a good colour and although she was sleepy, I felt much happier this time around than after her first operation.

In fact, it was only half an hour or so before she was sitting up and asking for a cup of tea, so I knew that all was well recovery wise. The difference between this procedure and her first operation was stark in terms of how she responded, though we knew there was still a long road ahead.

The next couple of days were spent watching the monitor that was attached to the probe in her head and seeing how it moved when she stood up, lay down, coughed etc. The fascination of this was a welcome distraction from the worry of what could be coming next.

After forty-eight hours of monitoring, Joanne was told by the medical team that her tonsils had slumped, her Chiari malformation had returned, and she would need another operation.

We were devastated and both had a lot of questions and concerns.

It was arranged for Joanne to go down to the clinic the next day to see the Consultant and review the scans.

When we saw the Consultant, we asked how this had happened and moreover, what could be done? And would it fail again?

The Consultant was great, he put us both at ease and explained he had been cautious in June with his approach and how much of the skull bone he'd removed. Jo's case, he reiterated, was one of the worst he had ever seen and couldn't believe how much pressure her tonsils had been under when they opened her up. His next comment I will never forget.

He was, he said, surprised that Joanne was still here.

The first operation, it transpired, they'd removed as little tonsil and skull as they thought they could get away with because he had wanted to be cautious. Once any of the skull and tonsils were removed, he explained, it wasn't possible to 'stick them back on'. This time the plan was to remove more and insert a titanium plate to prevent any further slump of Joanne's tonsils. This would also help to restore and keep the free flow of CSF (cerebral spinal fluid).

I asked him if it was a risky operation for Joanne given what happened to her the first time and was reassured that although it was a tricky operation, there would be two consultant surgeons present (apparently the norm for a redo). They were also planning to insert an NG tube whilst she was under which would remain in situ until they were happy with her swallow reflex.

It sounded as if they had considered every eventuality, but I remember Joanne asking that given the risks, should she just be happy with the state she was in now? She could watch TV and converse with family and friends for short periods of time, she said, and was she selfish for wanting more?

Joanne is one of the most selfless people I've ever met, so for her to even be considering not having the operation for risk of being selfish, was mind blowing. I have never been prouder of her, which was echoed by the consultant who told her how brave and resilient she was. He was confident this operation would provide her with a much better state of living. One word of warning though – this operation was going to be more complicated, so we were to expect a rougher recovery and for Joanne to be in hospital for 10-14 days.

The redo operation was, in the end, delayed quite some time since the wound on her head from the ICP probe became infected. It was frustrating waiting for this to heal and for a date for her redo to be organised. The secretary at the neurocentre was brilliant, though. She was so patient with Joanne whenever she had any questions or queries, and the two of them built up a lovely rapport.

This is actually a great tip - get to know the secretary and stay on their good side. It helped us no end.

Eventually the wound healed, and we had an appointment with the consultants to check we were all in agreement to go ahead. Joanne was still in two minds, but when she met with the consultants and told them how she was on a day-to-day basis, they reassured her that a redo was the way to go, and they were confident they could improve her life to some degree.

I feel that this helped us both so much, to hear their confidence and be reassured by them, and it took away the need to question whetherto have the operation or not. It did not make operation day any easier, though.

I went to work that day as I knew I would need time off after the operation to be with Jo. I spoke to her on the phone first thing, and she sounded remarkably calm. I knew she was now at peace with her decision and that it was the best option for her.

As soon as I finished work, I headed over to the neurocentre to visit. She looked so much better than after the first operation. Yes, she still had an NG tube in, but she was talking and sounding normal, not gurgly and wet like last time.

The next couple of days followed a similar pattern to the first operation though, where she had an awful day crying in pain and feeling sick, and then a day where she just slept. But I was happy to leave her at night this time. She was different. It all felt different.

I think it was day five when her dad went to visit whilst I took one of our sons back to university. I couldn't believe it when I had a phone call to say she had been discharged! I wasn't ready – nothing was prepared for her at home. They'd told us in the clinic and at the pre-op stage she would be in hospital for 10-14 days, so how come she was being discharged so early? She didn't even have a bag or case with her to bring home her belongings.

I was concerned they were rushing it, so I rang the ward and asked to speak to the nurse in charge of her care. They reassured me that the team were more than happy with Joanne's progress, she had done so well and was fine to go home. Even though I insisted I had nothing sorted for her they reassured me that home would now be the best place for Joanne to recover.

Once home, Joanne recovered steadily and at a good pace until she got to where we are at today.

Now, day to day life is very hard. Jo's window of what she can do is very limited.

I know I must be the one who says, 'yes you can do that', or 'no, you can't', and Jo is very stubborn. But I know her so well. I can see it in her face, in her body language when she's tired – sometimes before she feels it herself.

One thing I have learned is that you have to know your partner better than you thought you would ever have to know them, and you need to build a level of trust that allows you to tell them that they simply cannot do something at that precise time.

There are advantages though. Joanne now can't go wandering round the shops on her own which is great for our finances!

But I jest. Any positives are far outweighed by the disadvantages of her condition.

It has changed us; we have had to shift the dynamics of our marriage. I do most of the cooking and the cleaning. Jo can struggle and cook a basic meal but then she's too tired to eat it, so there's just no point.

I've had to learn how external factors can affect her too. It could be the weather or the environment and it's hard, if ever she's poorly, to know if it's the Chiari affecting her or something more simple, like a common cold.

Joanne was always very strong willed and independent, and it has been so hard to see her lose this. I think in many ways, this has been the toughest pill to swallow of it all.

But we've learned to worry about different things now and we no longer sweat the small stuff.

Chiari has affected our whole family.

It's Joanne's illness, but it's our fight and we are stronger now than we've ever been.

She is incredible.

And of my wife, I could not be more proud.

The End

(Resource Pages follow)

JOANNE ROBERTSON

***

Resources

***

Suggested List for your Hospital Stay

- Pyjamas that fasten up the front rather than those that go over your head
- Dressing gown
- Slippers
- Toiletries (Toothbrush, Deodorant etc)
- Dry shampoo (useful for freshening your hair until you are allowed to fully wash it)
- Facial wipes or baby wipes - great for freshening up until you can have a shower
- Lip balm - lips may get dry when wearing a mask
- Earplugs
- Eye mask - I found neurological wards to be incredibly bright
- Long charging cable for your mobile phone
- Headphones so that you can watch things on your phone, the television or just to shut your eyes and pretend you're resting when you want some peace and quiet
- Notebook and pen - to write things down as you remember them and give a list to your loved ones of what to bring when they next visit
- Magazines - you probably won't feel up to reading a book so magazines are great
- Loose change for the sweet trolley
- Plain or ginger biscuits to help with nausea

Useful Contacts

Ann Conroy Trust

www.annconroytrust.org

Tel: 0300 111 0004

email: info@annconroytrust.org

Chiari Malformation Groups on Facebook

www.facebook.com/chiarimalformationuk

www.facebook.com/groups/ChiariGroupBSF

Has Your Child been diagnosed with Chiari?

Conquer Chiara, US Charity:

https://tinyurl.com/y55y7y7b

Chiari Type 1 Malformation For Parents:

https://kidshealth.org/en/parents/chiari.html

Online Resource: Chiari Malformation (Brain and Spine Foundation Booklet)

https://tinyurl.com/ydgocl32

https://www.brainandspine.org.uk/our-publications/booklets/chiari-malformation

Chiari Malformation (NHS Choices)

https://tinyurl.com/yc9xsdch

***

Notes

***

Notes

_____

_____

_____

_____

_____

_____

_____

_____

_____

_____

_____

_____

CPSIA information can be obtained
at www.ICGtesting.com
Printed in the USA
BVHW061411271221
624935BV00011B/379

9 780995 642461